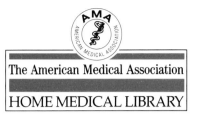

The American Medical Association

HOME MEDICAL LIBRARY

PRACTICAL
FAMILY
HEALTH

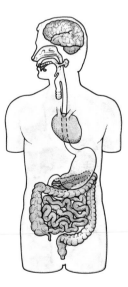

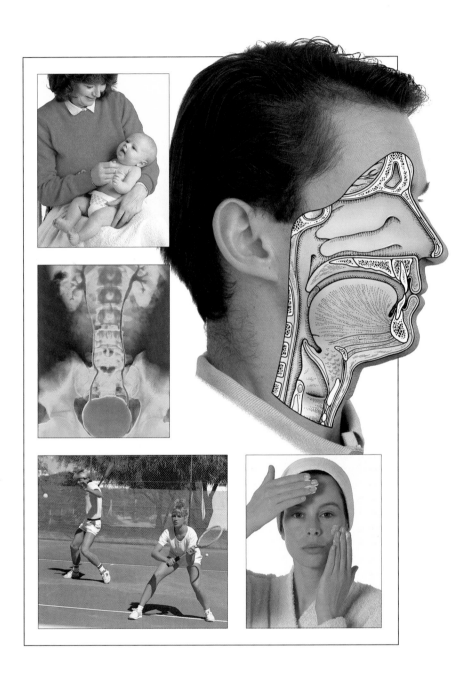

THE AMERICAN
MEDICAL ASSOCIATION

PRACTICAL
FAMILY
HEALTH

Medical Editor
CHARLES B. CLAYMAN, MD

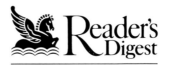

THE READER'S DIGEST ASSOCIATION, INC.
Pleasantville, New York/Montreal

The information in this book reflects current medical knowledge. The
recommendations and information are appropriate in most cases;
however, they are not a substitute for medical diagnosis. For specific
information concerning your personal medical condition, the AMA
suggests that you consult a physician.

The names of organizations, products, or alternative therapies appearing
in this book are given for informational purposes only. Their inclusion
does not imply AMA endorsement, nor does the omission of any
organization, product, or alternative therapy indicate AMA disapproval.

The AMA Home Medical Library is distinct from and unrelated to the series
of health books published by Random House, Inc., in conjunction with the
American Medical Association under the names "The AMA Home
Reference Library" and "The AMA Home Health Library."

Library of Congress Cataloging in Publication Data

American Medical Association.
    Practical family health / the American Medical Association ;
medical editor, Charles B. Clayman.
      p. cm. — (The AMA home medical library)
    Includes index.
    ISBN 0-89577-335-X
    1. Medicine, Popular. 2. Health. 3. First aid in illness and
injury. I. Clayman, Charles B. II. Title. III. Series: American
Medical Association. AMA home medical library.
RC81.A542 1989
613 — dc20   89-8464
                                       CIP

FOREWORD

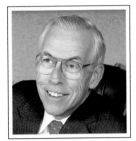

Good health is one of your most cherished possessions, but staying healthy is not just a matter of common sense. This volume of The AMA Home Medical Library is designed to give you the practical information you need both to maintain good health and cope with troublesome symptoms as they arise.

Over the last few decades, millions of Americans have learned the benefits of preventing illness through an active, healthy life-style. This change in attitude has led to a significant decrease in the rate of coronary heart disease and an increase in overall life expectancy. In the first chapter of this volume, we concentrate on what has been called the anticoronary life-style. We hope that you and members of your family will follow the advice on diet, exercise, managing stress, and the importance of having regular medical checkups.

Of course, some of us will continue to feel sick from time to time. Our chapter on health problems shows you how to tackle the most common symptoms and gives practical advice on when to call your doctor for guidance. The remaining chapters address the subjects of body maintenance, home nursing, and first aid. People today want clear, reliable, and up-to-date advice on these important topics. For each section there are instructions in an easy-to-understand format.

Bookstores are overflowing with health books promoting all kinds of diets, exercises, treatments, and theories. This volume does not contain "breakthrough" advice of that kind. Instead, it sets out in plain English the medical facts — the information gathered by careful scientific research. Medical science cannot prolong life indefinitely and does not attempt to do so. What it can do is help more people remain in good health right up to the end of their full, natural life span.

We at the American Medical Association wish you and your family the best of health.

JAMES S. TODD, MD
Executive Vice President
American Medical Association

CONTENTS

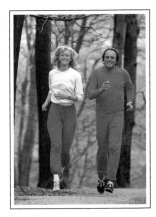

CHAPTER ONE

HEALTH FOR A LIFETIME

MAINTAINING yourself and your family in a state of good health rests on the same principles that keep your house or automobile in good condition. That means prevention rather than repair – both primary prevention, which consists of following a health-promoting life-style, and secondary prevention, which involves detecting and treating the warning signs of future trouble.

This chapter starts with a simple questionnaire that will help you decide whether you are making the right choices for your health. It will also help you identify the aspects of your lifestyle that may need attention. It is all too easy to push to the back of your mind any concerns about nagging symptoms, or to postpone doing something about smoking or medical checkups on the grounds that "I'm too busy right now to be bothered with that." But remember that your health should be a top priority; without good health you are less likely to achieve your goals at work and hopes for your family. The next two sections emphasize the positive aspects of exercise and diet. There's little point in exercising every day if you don't enjoy it. If you find some form of exercise that gives you pleasure, you will be more likely to do it regularly. You'll also

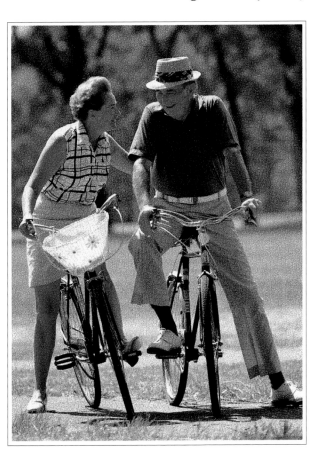

learn how much better you feel when you are in good physical condition. The same principles hold true with your diet. With the exception of a few basic rules, like cutting down on saturated fats, worrying about what *not* to eat does little good. It is more useful to model your family's diet on a variety of appetizing and health-promoting foods. If the food tastes good – and it's good for you – you'll continue to eat it.

Our section on hazards to health is concerned mainly with correcting false beliefs. Many people spend time worrying about air pollution or food additives when, statistically, the *real* dangers for many Americans stem from smoking, being overweight, consuming too much alcohol, and, particularly for those under the age of 40, from traffic accidents and the ownership of firearms. These risks can all be substantially reduced by attention to life-style.

Finally, no matter how healthy your lifestyle, you may have inherited a tendency to a disease. As explained in our section on monitoring family health, each of us can benefit from the wide range of screening techniques that are now available for detecting disease. Early treatment of any condition is much more likely to bring about a successful cure, and is usually simpler and less expensive in the long run.

SEVEN CHOICES FOR HEALTH

Everyone has at least some control over his or her future health. The decisions that you make both early in life and later on can have a significant influence on your physical and mental well-being.

Answer this questionnaire and see how you score. Remember that, when it comes to health, a positive score in some places does not mean that you can allow yourself a negative score in others. If you really want to be healthy, an honest YES is the answer you should be giving. And, if your answer is NO, it is never too late to make a change for the better in your life-style.

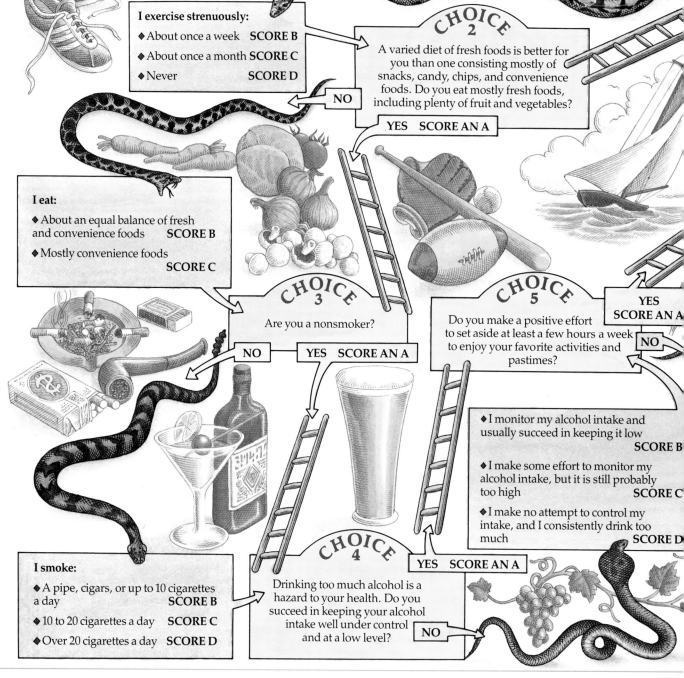

I exercise strenuously:
◆ About once a week **SCORE B**
◆ About once a month **SCORE C**
◆ Never **SCORE D**

CHOICE 2
A varied diet of fresh foods is better for you than one consisting mostly of snacks, candy, chips, and convenience foods. Do you eat mostly fresh foods, including plenty of fruit and vegetables?
YES SCORE AN A
NO

I eat:
◆ About an equal balance of fresh and convenience foods **SCORE B**
◆ Mostly convenience foods **SCORE C**

CHOICE 3
Are you a nonsmoker?
NO   YES SCORE AN A

CHOICE 5
Do you make a positive effort to set aside at least a few hours a week to enjoy your favorite activities and pastimes?
YES SCORE AN A
NO

◆ I monitor my alcohol intake and usually succeed in keeping it low **SCORE B**
◆ I make some effort to monitor my alcohol intake, but it is still probably too high **SCORE C**
◆ I make no attempt to control my intake, and I consistently drink too much **SCORE D**

I smoke:
◆ A pipe, cigars, or up to 10 cigarettes a day **SCORE B**
◆ 10 to 20 cigarettes a day **SCORE C**
◆ Over 20 cigarettes a day **SCORE D**

CHOICE 4
Drinking too much alcohol is a hazard to your health. Do you succeed in keeping your alcohol intake well under control and at a low level?
YES SCORE AN A
NO

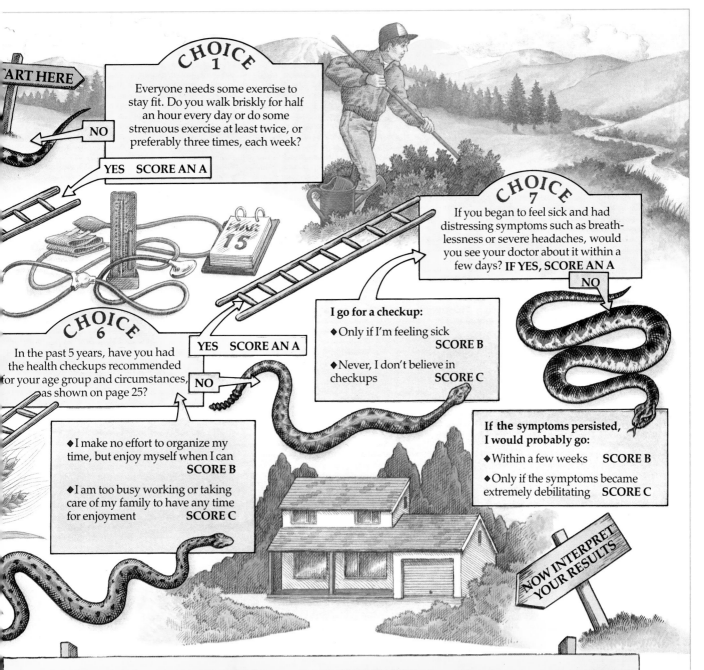

CHOICE 1
Everyone needs some exercise to stay fit. Do you walk briskly for half an hour every day or do some strenuous exercise at least twice, or preferably three times, each week?

START HERE

NO

YES   SCORE AN A

CHOICE 7
If you began to feel sick and had distressing symptoms such as breathlessness or severe headaches, would you see your doctor about it within a few days? **IF YES, SCORE AN A**

NO

I go for a checkup:
- Only if I'm feeling sick   **SCORE B**
- Never, I don't believe in checkups   **SCORE C**

YES   SCORE AN A

CHOICE 6
In the past 5 years, have you had the health checkups recommended for your age group and circumstances, as shown on page 25?

NO

- I make no effort to organize my time, but enjoy myself when I can   **SCORE B**
- I am too busy working or taking care of my family to have any time for enjoyment   **SCORE C**

If the symptoms persisted, I would probably go:
- Within a few weeks   **SCORE B**
- Only if the symptoms became extremely debilitating   **SCORE C**

NOW INTERPRET YOUR RESULTS

HOW DID YOU SCORE?

Mostly As:
The choices you have made are directly benefiting your health and well-being.

Mostly Bs:
While your choices do not place you in immediate danger, there are ways you could begin to improve your health.

Mostly Cs:
Your choice of life-style is placing your health at risk.

One or more Ds:
Any D indicates that your health is being seriously undermined, regardless of any other efforts you are making to stay healthy. It should be your first priority to remove any D from your life-style.

A mixture of As, Bs, and Cs:
You are not playing a sufficiently active role in maintaining good health — try to aim for an A in all areas.

STAYING FIT

Why do you need to be fit? First, because regular exercise benefits every part of your body, helping it perform more efficiently and extending its trouble-free functioning into old age. If you exercise regularly you are likely to have lower levels of cholesterol in your blood and are less likely to develop high blood pressure or heart disease. Just as important, regular exercise enhances your vitality and sense of physical well-being, making you feel more relaxed and confident, improving the quality of your sleep, and helping you combat stress.

EXERCISE AND THE BODY

Not all exercise is of equal value to health. The type known as "aerobic" is the best exercise for increasing your general level of fitness, especially the performance of your heart and lungs. Aerobic exercise involves any continuous activity, such as jogging, cycling, rowing, or swimming, that makes you a little breathless, but which does not cause you to become out of breath and force you to stop.

During aerobic exercise the heart and lungs work harder, increasing the rate at which oxygen-rich blood is circulated around the body to the muscles. The oxygen combines with glucose in the muscle cells to supply the energy they need. Because there is sufficient oxygen, the cells tire slowly and the exercise can be continued for a long period.

Anaerobic exercise, on the other hand, consists of a short, sharp burst of strenuous effort, such as sprinting or lifting a heavy weight. The supply of oxygen to the muscles does not keep pace with the amount of oxygen the muscles need for their task. Lactic acid, a by-product of anaerobic chemical reactions, can build up in the muscle cells and cause pain by irritating them. The overall effect of repeated anaerobic exercise is to increase

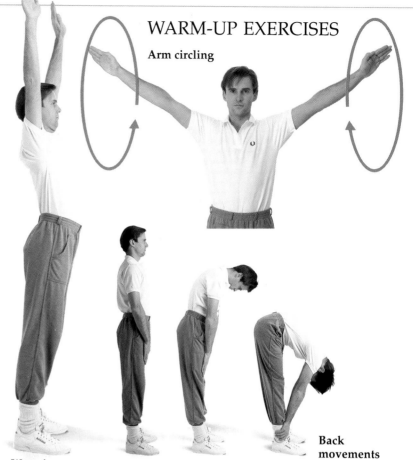

WARM-UP EXERCISES

Arm circling

Back movements

Warming up

Always warm up for 10 minutes before strenuous activity with a program of exercises. Arm circling, bending and straightening back movements, leg swinging, and side-to-side shoulder stretches will exercise the main muscle groups. A warm-up increases the blood flow through your tissues and makes them more elastic, reducing the risk of injury.

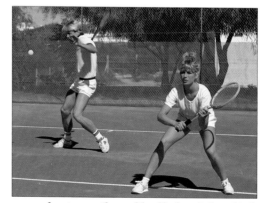

Playing tennis
Tennis is a stimulating competitive game (left) that involves periods of intense effort during which there is much anaerobic production of energy in the muscles. The resultant buildup of lactic acid may cause considerable pain and stiffness for anyone out of condition, making tennis a game better suited for people wanting to stay fit than those getting in shape.

muscle strength and bulk, but it has little effect on the heart and lungs.

To minimize muscle pain, always begin with a warm-up program before exercise. Cool down afterward by repeating your warm-up muscle stretches or by continuing to walk, cycle, row, or swim slowly for a few minutes.

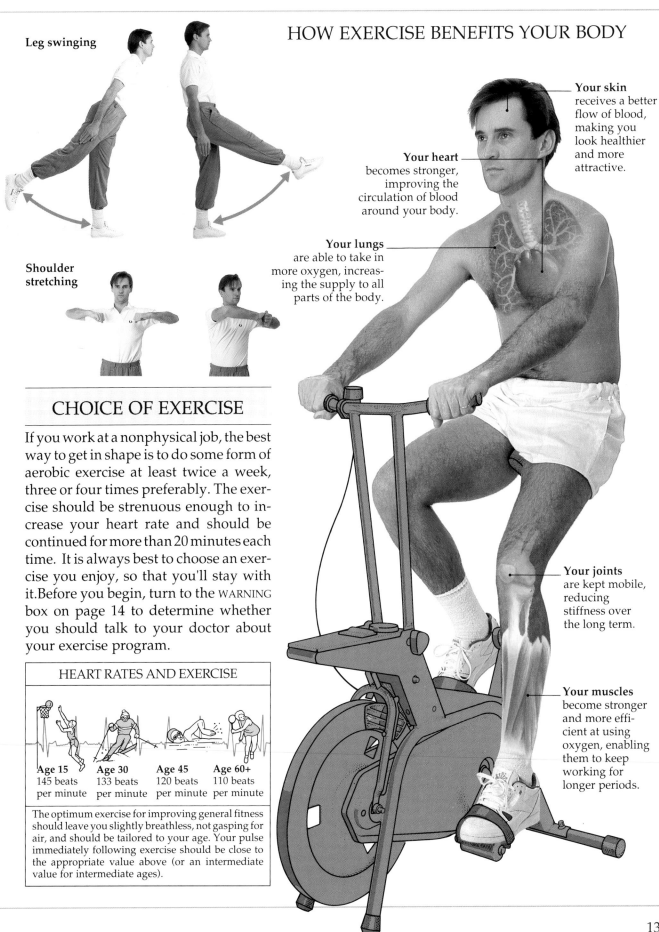

Leg swinging

HOW EXERCISE BENEFITS YOUR BODY

Your skin
receives a better flow of blood, making you look healthier and more attractive.

Your heart
becomes stronger, improving the circulation of blood around your body.

Your lungs
are able to take in more oxygen, increasing the supply to all parts of the body.

Shoulder stretching

Your joints
are kept mobile, reducing stiffness over the long term.

Your muscles
become stronger and more efficient at using oxygen, enabling them to keep working for longer periods.

CHOICE OF EXERCISE

If you work at a nonphysical job, the best way to get in shape is to do some form of aerobic exercise at least twice a week, three or four times preferably. The exercise should be strenuous enough to increase your heart rate and should be continued for more than 20 minutes each time. It is always best to choose an exercise you enjoy, so that you'll stay with it.Before you begin, turn to the WARNING box on page 14 to determine whether you should talk to your doctor about your exercise program.

HEART RATES AND EXERCISE

Age 15
145 beats per minute

Age 30
133 beats per minute

Age 45
120 beats per minute

Age 60+
110 beats per minute

The optimum exercise for improving general fitness should leave you slightly breathless, not gasping for air, and should be tailored to your age. Your pulse immediately following exercise should be close to the appropriate value above (or an intermediate value for intermediate ages).

ASK YOUR DOCTOR
STAYING FIT

Q **I have been warned that jogging regularly may do more harm than good. What are the real facts about jogging?**

A Jogging is an excellent way of exercising to improve your fitness. Any harm from jogging comes from failing to warm up properly, wearing unsuitable footwear or clothing, running long distances on hard or uneven ground, or trying to do too much before you are fully fit.

Q **My elderly mother insists on climbing the stairs rather than taking the elevator. Does this count as exercise, and is it good for her?**

A Climbing stairs is a good form of exercise for healthy people because it gets the heart, lungs, and muscles working. However, it can place strain on the hips, ankles, and especially the knees, so if your mother suffers from arthritis, stair-climbing may aggravate the pain, stiffness, and swelling in those joints. Anyone with a heart or lung disorder, such as angina or emphysema, should try to avoid stairs if climbing them brings on chest pains or severe breathlessness.

Q **If I'm not feeling well, should I suspend my normal exercise routine until I'm better?**

A You should avoid strenuous exercise because it may make your condition worse. Strenuous exercise during an infection, such as influenza or cystitis, may be detrimental to the heart muscle, resulting in chest pain and, occasionally, a reduction in the heart's efficiency. You should also rest if you have a fever, a cough, or swollen glands.

Getting started

Many people make the mistake of trying to do too much exercise too soon. The best approach is to build up your routine gradually. If you have not done any exercise for some time, you might want to begin with a brisk walk around the block. When you can cover a couple of miles without any difficulty, you can

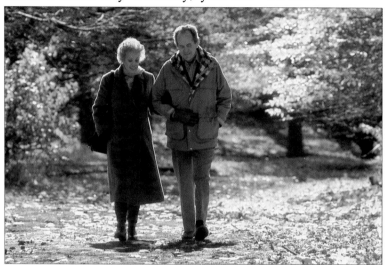

Enjoying a walk
Walking briskly in the open air stimulates the heart, lungs, muscles, and mind.

increase your distance and the number of times you walk each week. You should adopt the same gradual approach to whatever exercise you choose – swimming, tennis, and so on. In middle age, it is wise to ask your doctor if you need any special exercise tests.

Whatever type of exercise you choose, it should make you feel tired, not totally exhausted. Although you can expect some stiffness over the first few days, it should not be severe. If you do too much, the resultant pain and exhaustion will sap your motivation to continue.

Exercise for a lifetime

As you grow older, regular exercise helps maintain the normal functioning of your joints, muscles, tendons, ligaments, and bones. Your joints will stay mobile and your muscle strength, balance, and coordination will be maintained. Freedom of movement and confidence in your body are valuable assets that need not be sacrificed with advancing years.

WARNING

Inform your doctor before starting an exercise program if you are overweight, a smoker, have a family history of heart disease, are over 35, or if you are suffering from any medical disorder.
  You should also be aware of certain symptoms during exercise that could be caused by excessive strain on your heart. They are:
♦ Chest pain
♦ Pain in your neck or arms
♦ Palpitations
♦ Severe breathlessness
♦ Feeling faint
If these symptoms occur, stop exercising and see your doctor.

EATING WELL

Eating is one of life's pleasures, yet many people feel guilty when they admit to enjoying their meals, believing that there must be something unhealthy, or even immoral, in their pleasure. This is nonsense. Of course, overeating that leads to obesity is dangerous to your health, but so, too, is extreme thinness.

You can determine whether your weight is right for your height by referring to the weight charts on page 108. Provided your weight is steady and within the recommended limits, the energy content (calories) in your food is balancing your energy output. Weigh yourself weekly; if your weight is more than 20 percent above what is recommended, or if you are gaining weight, then you are eating too much.

Always look for fresh foods, which have a higher nutritional value. Foods that are salted, smoked, cured, processed, or preserved may contain additives or toxic substances that are hazardous to health. They are less advisable, as are foods with a high refined sugar content.

DIET AND NUTRITION

Nutritionists have identified six important elements that are indispensable for maintaining a balanced diet:

♦ **Carbohydrate** – best eaten in high-fiber form in raw or lightly cooked vegetables, brown rice, and whole-grain cereal products – should provide 50 to 60 percent of the energy that your body needs to perform efficiently.

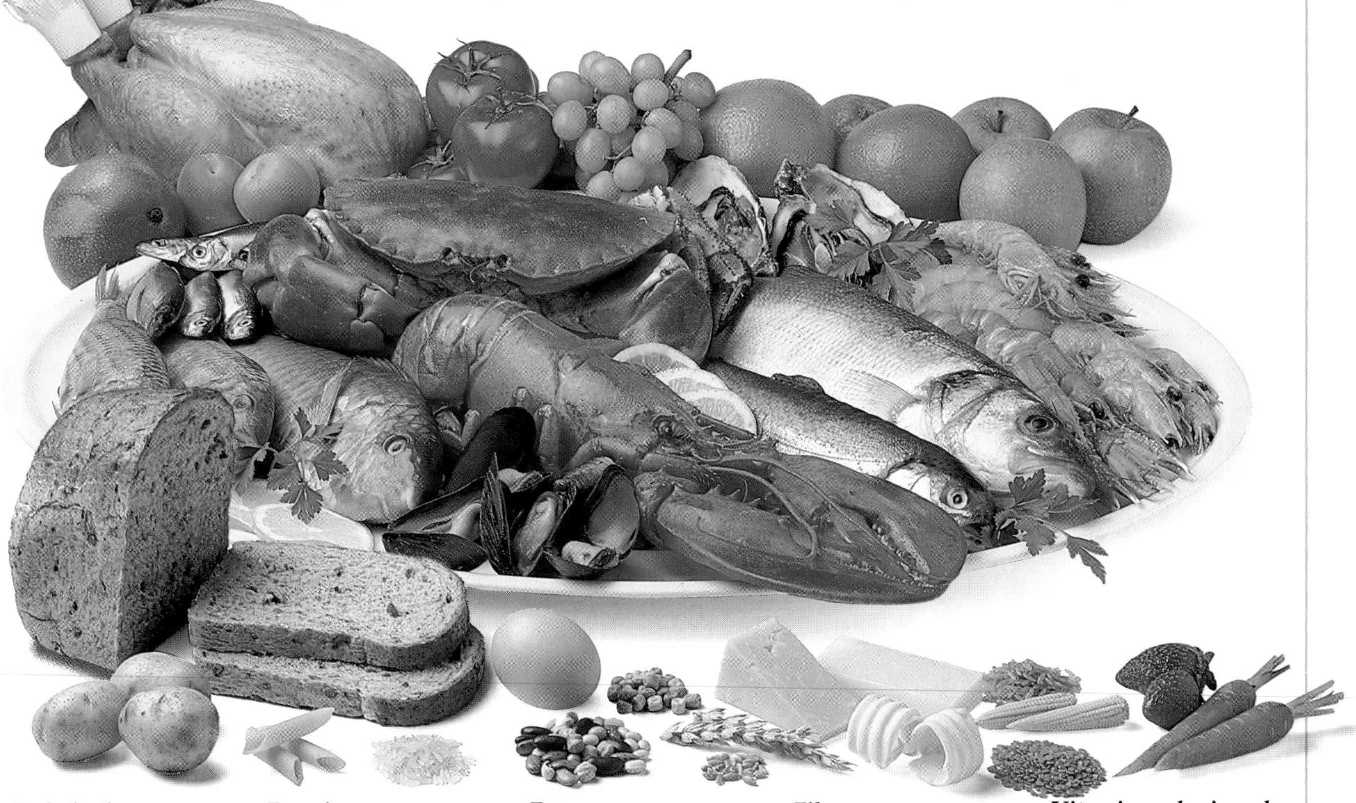

Carbohydrate sources
Bread, cereals, flour, pasta, rice, potatoes, peas, beans, lentils, and nuts. All seeds contain carbohydrate.

Protein sources
Lean meat and poultry, eggs, fish, seafood, low-fat milk, peas, beans, cereals, and potatoes.

Fat sources
Margarine, butter, cream, yogurt, cheese, vegetable and fish oils, animal fat, egg yolks, and lard.

Fiber sources
Peas, beans, whole-grain cereals and bread, brown rice, and raw or lightly cooked fruit and vegetables.

Vitamin and mineral sources
Fresh fruit and vegetables, fish, whole-grain cereals, dairy products, and liver.

VITAMIN SUPPLEMENTS

Should people take regular doses of multivitamins as a precaution against vitamin deficiency?

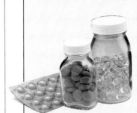

Nutritionists say no. Vitamins are like engine oil for an automobile. Too little is damaging, but too much may also be harmful.

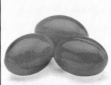

It is more important that your diet contains a balanced proportion of vitamins and minerals. Fresh vegetables and fruit contain large amounts of vitamins, especially A and C.

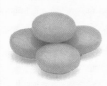

Thus, a teenager who eats mostly candies, chips, french fries, hot dogs, and other processed foods may be vitamin-deficient. However, the answer lies in improving the diet, not in adding a vitamin pill.

♦ **Protein** is needed by your body for growth, repair, and replacement of muscle and other body tissues. Your protein intake should include lean meat eaten no more than once a day.

♦ **Fat** provides energy, but intake of saturated fats should be limited (see CHOLESTEROL AND YOUR HEART on page 17). No more than 30 percent of energy should come from fat. The average American eats a diet in which fat accounts for more than 35 percent of the total energy gained.

♦ **Fiber** in the diet helps the human digestive system to work optimally. A substantial amount of indigestible fiber is needed. Foods such as fresh fruits and vegetables, whole-grain bread, and brown rice provide much more fiber than the processed equivalents.

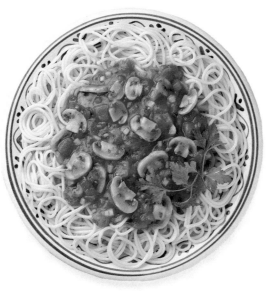

♦ **Vitamins** – complex chemicals that the body cannot make for itself but which are essential for the functioning of nerves, muscles, skin, and bone – are required in small amounts. In all, the body needs about a dozen or so different vitamins.

♦ **Minerals** such as calcium for the bones, iodine for thyroid function, and iron for the blood must also be provided by your diet. A balanced diet contains all the minerals that your body needs.

THE WORLD'S HEALTHIEST DIETS

The nations in which eating and cooking are given a high priority as important features of social and business life, notably France, Italy, Indonesia, and China, have cuisines that positively promote health. By contrast, our own fast-food culture promotes high rates of disease that is related to diet.

Why are the Mediterranean and Pacific cuisines praised by nutritionists and physicians? First, the sources of protein include a lot of fish, including shellfish, squid, and octopus. Meat is likely to be lean chicken, goat, or veal. What these protein sources have in common is a low proportion of fat. Furthermore, the

Low-fat cuisine
As long as no cheese, fatty meat, or animal fats are used, a pasta (left) or stir-fry dish (below) contains little saturated fat.

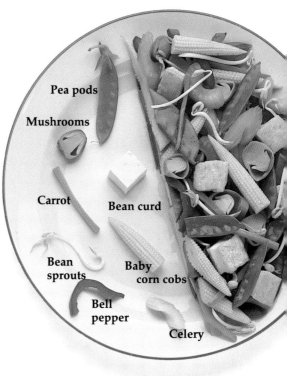

Pea pods

Mushrooms

Carrot

Bean curd

Bean sprouts

Baby corn cobs

Bell pepper

Celery

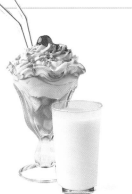

protein is usually mixed with a carbohydrate, such as rice or pasta. The result is that the dishes contain optimum proportions of fat, protein, and carbohydrate, ensuring that the body is able to gain the energy it requires from the most appropriate source.

Second, little of the fat content comes from milk, butter, and lard. Cooking is done mostly in vegetable oils; olive oil is also used in salad dressings and mayonnaise, and as a source of flavor and moisture for bread. Little of the carbohydrate in these diets comes in the form of refined sugar. Instead, rice, beans, potatoes, and lentils, which have the bonus of including substantial quantities of fiber, are eaten. Fruit and vegetables make a large contribution to the total energy content; they are rich in vitamins, and they contain useful fiber.

CHOLESTEROL AND YOUR HEART

The central idea behind most medical advice concerning diet is that good health requires a low level of fats and cholesterol in the blood. Research studies have shown repeatedly that people with high cholesterol levels are more likely to suffer heart attacks, strokes, and other diseases of the blood vessels.

The link with heart disease is easy to understand. The underlying cause of most heart attacks and strokes is atherosclerosis, a narrowing of the blood vessels caused by deposits of a yellow, greasy substance called atheroma on the inside lining of the arteries. Atheroma (from the Greek word for porridge) consists mainly of cholesterol, which is an essential part of the structure of cell walls. However, when there is too much cholesterol in the blood, it accumulates in the walls of blood vessels, narrowing them and decreasing the vital blood flow to the heart and brain.

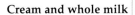

Cream and whole milk

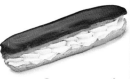

Creamy pastries

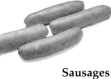

Sausages

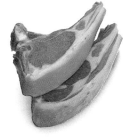

Salami

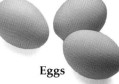

Eggs

Which fats can be harmful?

Fats that are solid in a cool kitchen – butter, lard, the fat on pork or lamb chops, or fat in beef joints – push up the cholesterol levels most easily. These fats are called saturated fats. Fats that are liquid or semiliquid – olive oil, vegetable oils, fish oils, and liquid margarines – are less harmful; these are unsaturated fats.

The simple message is: eat less fat. When you do use fat, choose unsaturated fats and select lean cuts of meat. This is a message that has helped to cut deaths from heart disease in the US from 286 per 100,000 in 1960 to 183 per 100,000 in 1984, a significant reduction.

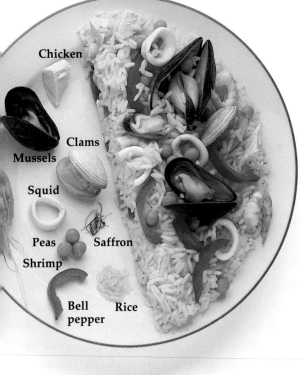

Chicken

Clams

Mussels

Squid

Peas Saffron

Shrimp

Bell   Rice
pepper

Spanish paella
Fresh seafood and vegetables make this traditional Mediterranean dish (above) a rich source of the nutrients that the body needs.

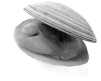

Cuts of fatty meat

Cutting down on fat
To guard against diseases of the heart and circulation, foods with a high fat content, such as those shown above, should be eaten only sparingly. Only one or two eggs should be eaten per week.

AVOIDING HEALTH HAZARDS

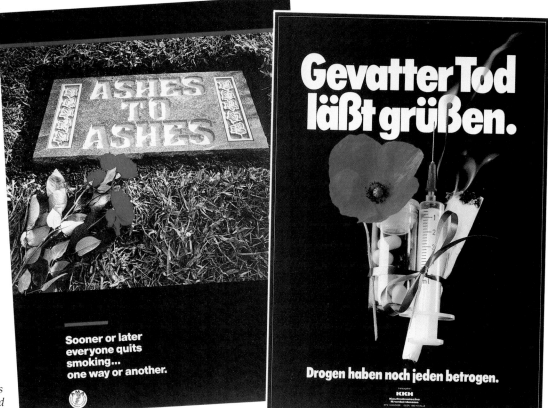

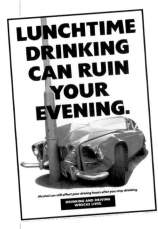

Risks to your life
Health organizations throughout the world are mounting increasingly direct campaigns to communicate the potentially lethal dangers of smoking (above right), drug abuse (far right), and driving while under the influence of alcohol (below).

What precautions can you take to stay healthy well into old age? Many people have a fatalistic attitude about their health, believing that, "If an accident doesn't get me, some disease will, regardless of what I do." However, a look at the statistics for the causes of death in the US makes it abundantly clear that your fate is not entirely "in the lap of the gods." There are several important choices you can make to protect yourself against potential sources of harm.

CAUSES OF DEATH

Up to the age of 44, injury is the leading cause of death and disability in the US. Motor vehicle accidents cause about 35,000 deaths each year in this age group,

and violent homicides account for about 12,000 deaths, most caused by gunshot wounds. There are 12,000 suicides, half of which are committed with firearms, making suicide the third main cause of death in young people.

What can be done?

There are several ways in which these alarming figures can be reduced. First, wearing seat belts has been shown conclusively to reduce the risk of death or serious injury for the drivers and passengers of motor vehicles; for motorcyclists and horseback riders, protective headgear is just as important. Second, alcohol is an important factor in traffic accidents and violence, and half of the 5,000 or so drownings a year in the US

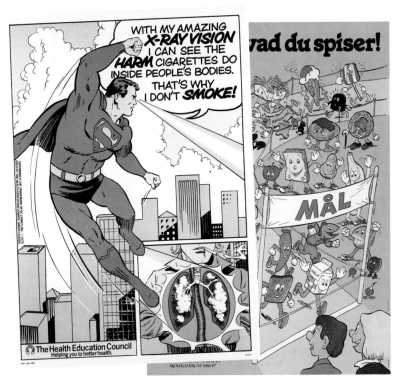

The Health Education Council
Helping you to better health.

smoking, maintain a low-fat diet that also keeps your weight in the normal range, and control any rise in blood pressure. By following this advice, Americans have reduced their death rate from heart disease by about one third in the past 25 years. However, it remains the leading cause of premature death.

Hazards after 65

After the age of 65, heart disease remains a major killer, but strokes cause as many deaths as heart disease between the ages of 60 and 80; after the age of 80, strokes cause twice as many deaths. Cancers are also a very important cause of disability and death for people older than 65. Even as we age, some deaths are avoidable, notably the cancers that are associated with smoking and excess alcohol consumption, and the strokes that are attributable to undetected or untreated high blood pressure.

SMOKING

Without doubt the single most important measure to improve both health and life expectancy in the US would be the elimination of tobacco smoking. In people younger than 65, the overall death rate is twice as high in smokers as it is in the nonsmoking population. Smoking is the main cause of lung cancer; it is a major contributor to premature deaths from heart disease (about 90 percent of deaths from heart attacks in people

are alcohol-related. Alcohol should not be consumed by anyone intending to drive or swim. Third, the involvement of firearms in more than 30,000 deaths of all ages annually has its own message: do not keep a firearm at home. Most of these deaths were either suicides or the result of domestic quarrels; those who died were victims of their own weapons. If you choose to own firearms for hunting, make sure they are locked securely in a suitable storage cabinet.

Taking care of your heart

After the age of 45, the dominant cause of death is heart disease. Research scientists still cannot explain fully the spectacular rise in the frequency of heart disease in the 20th century. One American man in five develops symptoms of heart disease by the age of 60. Between the ages of 40 and 60, deaths from this condition outnumber those from stroke, bronchitis, and cancers of the lung, stomach, and breast combined.

The prevention of coronary heart disease is now the primary message from health and medical groups. Their advice for an anticoronary life-style is: give up

Warning the children
By expressing ideas in amusing, colorful sketches (above) and by using popular figures such as Superman (above left), health educators can convey information and warnings to children in terms that they can understand.

Safety at home
A firearm kept at home is always a potential hazard to the owner. The British campaign poster below illustrates one risk, but there are also many deaths due to firearm accidents.

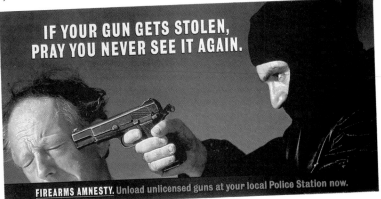

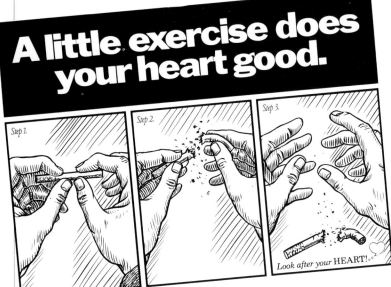

A little exercise does your heart good.

Step 1.

Step 2.

Step 3.

Look after your HEART!

Getting the message across
As illustrated above and below, pointed observation is being used with increasing effect in health education.

younger than 50 are in cigarette smokers); and it is an important factor in cancers of the mouth, tongue, lip, larynx, esophagus, bladder, and cervix.

In addition, smokers damage their lungs and skin. The decline in lung function that occurs with age progresses more rapidly in smokers, as does wrinkling of the skin. Smoking is the main cause of chronic bronchitis. A smoker's cough is, in fact, evidence of chronic irritation of the lungs.

Breaking the habit

When you stop smoking, you automatically reduce your chances of dying from a smoking-related disease. The longer you abstain, the less likely you are to die from a smoking-related disease. After about 15 years of not smoking, your chances of early death are about the same as those of a lifelong nonsmoker. Moreover, the length of time you smoked makes little difference in this general trend, so it is always worth quitting. The average smoker's chances of dying of lung cancer (compared to those of a nonsmoker) decrease from the time he or she stops smoking. This tendency also applies to other smoking-related illnesses.

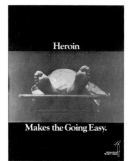

Heroin

Makes the Going Easy.

Drugs
Drugs other than alcohol vary in their immediate and long-term effects, but the outstanding problem associated with their abuse is that of dependence. Abuse of heroin, cocaine, morphine, or opium leads rapidly to addiction. Anti-anxiety drugs and barbiturates tend to result in addiction in the longer term. Drug dependence is a disease that, without treatment, usually worsens with time. Professional medical help should be sought immediately if a family member has a drug addiction problem.

ALCOHOL

There are three main reasons society is concerned about excessive drinking. First, alcohol consumption is an important factor in accidents on the road, at work, and in the home; it often precipitates domestic and other violence, marital problems, and divorce; and it impairs work performance. Second, alcohol can damage the heart, liver, nervous system, and brain, among other organ systems. It increases the chances of the development of cancer of the larynx, the esophagus, and the pancreas. And third, a substantial fraction of heavy drinkers are suffering from unrecognized early alcohol dependency, often with disastrous effects on their mental and physical health and personal relationships.

Knowing your limits

Using the guide to the alcoholic content of drinks below, try to keep your intake as low as possible. If you are a woman who is pregnant or planning to have a baby soon, abstain from alcohol altogether. Also abstain if you are planning to drive or operate machinery.

DRINKS CONTAINING EQUAL AMOUNTS OF ALCOHOL

No alcoholic drinks are "safer" than others. As a guide, the three examples shown here contain the same amount of alcohol.

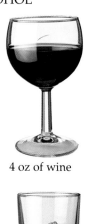

4 oz of wine

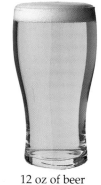

12 oz of beer

1.5 oz of hard liquor

MANAGING STRESS

Stress is a fact of life that carries both good and bad aspects. The stress experienced by a rock climber, a race-car driver, or a stage performer may be exhilarating and life-enhancing. But, for many people, stress means a state of almost continuous, and unwanted, tension and apprehension that may eventually lead to chronic anxiety, depression, physical symptoms, and illness. Fortunately, by monitoring stress levels and taking effective action early, these problems can usually be avoided.

The way in which you respond to stress depends partly on personality, partly on experience, and partly on the duration and kind of stress involved. Psychiatrists learned during World War II that combat troops could respond with courage and enthusiasm for several months, but after that even the toughest became battle-weary. The same is true in everyday life. A demanding job or a challenging sport may be stimulating at first, but, if the pressures are unrelenting, the individual may eventually begin to suffer. Ideally, the anxiety produced by stress should be a temporary condition that arises for a specific reason and subsides when the difficulty has been resolved. It is only when feelings of anxiety persist and come to dominate a person's life that they gradually become the cause of illness.

Stress factors
In the US, financial and work-related problems are the most frequently cited causes of stress, particularly among higher income groups. Two thirds of visits to a doctor are believed to be stress-related.

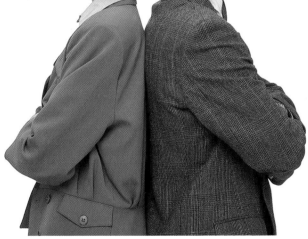

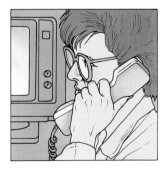

Stress at work
Change of job
Fear of unemployment

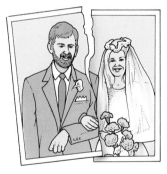
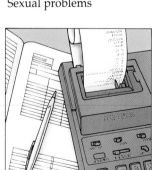
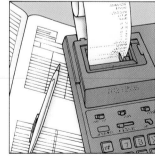

Family relationships
Separation and divorce
Sexual problems

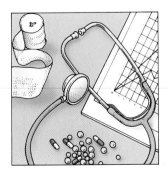

Family illness
Accidents
Bereavement

A crying baby
 or problem child
Child care

Home mortgage and upkeep
Insurance
Moving

Taxes
Medical insurance
College tuition

MONITORING STRESS

One way of measuring your stress level is to count the number of important life events or changes that you have undergone recently. High on the list of stressful events are bereavement, job changes or a promotion, any serious illness in the family, moving, marital difficulties, financial problems, or the imminent birth of a child. Most people can cope with one or two changes of this type without much problem – but three different stressful events may make life difficult, while four or more are generally more than anyone can cope with effectively.

Signs and symptoms

Another method is to be aware of physical clues. Our bodies are designed to respond to stress physically rather than mentally – a reaction known as the "fight or flight" response. This means that the human animal's reaction to a threat is either to fight or to run away. The preparation for these physical responses is for the heart to beat faster, the muscles to tense, the hair to stand on end, and the skin to sweat. If the threat is mental or emotional rather than physical, these same responses occur, but are inappropriate. Sweating palms and a rapid heart rate are not much help when you are required to give a speech.

In time, chronic anxiety may cause the bodily changes associated with stress to become more or less fixed. Symptoms such as frequent headaches, palpitations, indigestion, backache, and aggravated skin conditions are possible results. If you find you are suffering many physical symptoms that defy obvious medical explanation, it could be that you are suffering from too much stress.

What can be done?

If you or a member of your family feels under pressure, take action to manage the problem. First, the stressful factors must be identified and confronted. It is

EXERCISES FOR RELIEVING PHYSICAL TENSION

Muscles that have become tensed by stress can be relaxed by these simple exercises. When doing them, it is best to wear loose, comfortable clothing that allows you to move freely. Repeat the exercises, one after the other, for 8 to 10 minutes. Then lie totally limp for a few more minutes to complete the session.

1 Lie face up on the floor with your eyes closed and your arms flat at your sides.

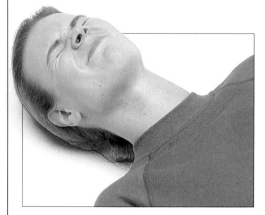

2 Tense your face muscles and then let them relax.

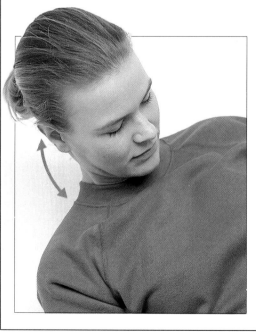

3 Lift your head and let it fall gently back. Keep your neck and jaw relaxed so that you can feel your throat opening.

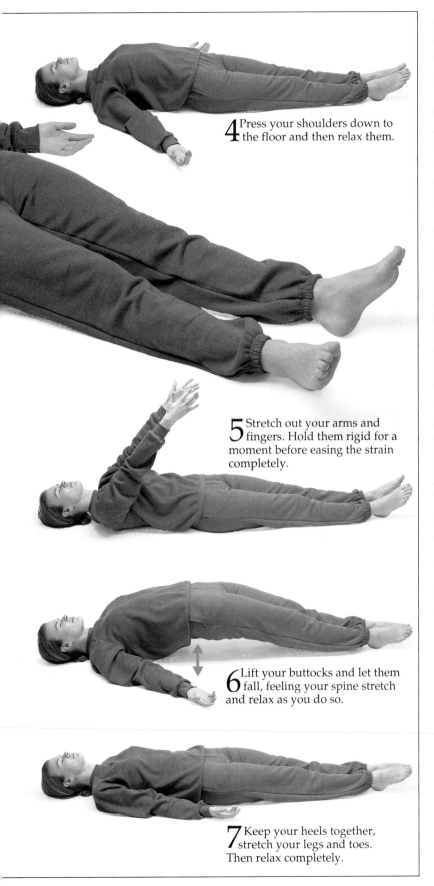

4 Press your shoulders down to the floor and then relax them.

5 Stretch out your arms and fingers. Hold them rigid for a moment before easing the strain completely.

6 Lift your buttocks and let them fall, feeling your spine stretch and relax as you do so.

7 Keep your heels together, stretch your legs and toes. Then relax completely.

usually helpful to talk frankly with those at the source of the problem, whether it is your spouse, your children, your parents, or your employer.

If your anxiety has resulted in physical symptoms or a mental condition such as depression, ask your doctor for advice. He or she may recommend a short course of medication, which is only the starting point for the recovery process rather than a solution in itself.

Perhaps most importantly, you may need to develop a new, more positive attitude to life and decision-making in which you concentrate on the present, identify the problems you are facing, make your decisions, and act promptly. Setting aside time for yourself, away from your work and your daily worries, is a good antidote to stress. Don't allow yourself to mope around brooding unproductively. Even if you feel "down," take a brisk walk around the block or find another activity that will give you pleasure and allow you to relax.

How to relieve tension

Inevitably, stress will cause you tension from time to time, but there are methods you can use to relax. Many of them can be done anywhere, anytime. You can try consciously to slow your breathing by taking deep, even breaths for 5 minutes whenever you feel the onset of tension. Or you can try a simple meditation method – just sit upright with your eyes closed in a quiet room and empty your mind of thoughts by concentrating on an image that has no emotional connotations. Gradually extend the meditation period from 5 minutes twice a day to 20 minutes at each session.

All forms of strenuous physical exercise help relieve tension caused by stress. In addition, the fatigue that follows strenuous exercise is conducive to sleeping soundly. You awake refreshed, alert, and better able to concentrate, all of which are useful in helping you respond to stress more effectively.

MONITORING FAMILY HEALTH

In the past, people believed that they needed to start worrying about their health only when they became sick. This attitude is outdated. Many important disorders–especially cancers–may pass unnoticed in the early stages. Symptoms then develop at a more advanced stage, by which time the disease is less likely to be treated successfully. Other conditions, such as high blood pressure, may never produce symptoms, but if left undetected can lead to serious health complications later in life.

Each of us should take responsibility for his or her own health and at least some responsibility for the health of our family. By arranging to have regular checkups, you can catch any potential problem early. Most people have their automobiles serviced at least once a year – surely your body, which must last a lifetime, deserves at least that much attention to its maintenance.

REGULAR SCREENING

Medical research has now established an optimum program of screening for the signs of potential disease. The program involves physical and instrumental examination of the body, along with laboratory tests on blood and urine. The frequency of the tests increases as you grow older, simply because diseases such as stroke and cancer are more common in old age. Recommended tests are shown in the chart on page 25. Further details on specific tests follow.

Testing blood pressure

Blood pressure is a measurement of the force with which blood is being pumped through your arteries. The pressure goes up when you are exercising or under stress, and falls during sleep and periods of relaxation. When your blood

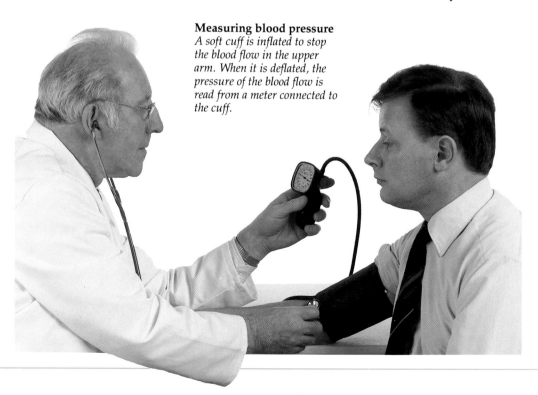

Measuring blood pressure
A soft cuff is inflated to stop the blood flow in the upper arm. When it is deflated, the pressure of the blood flow is read from a meter connected to the cuff.

HEALTH CHECKUPS YOU CAN DO AT HOME

TEST AND PURPOSE	FOR WHOM RECOMMENDED	WHEN AND HOW OFTEN
SKIN EXAMINATION To detect any new mole, or any mole that has begun to bleed, itch, or grow, that may be a sign of skin cancer.	Everyone should check his or her skin, but people who experience prolonged sun exposure should be rigorous in their checking.	All adults over the age of 20 should be checked during their regular physical examination.
BREAST EXAMINATION To detect any lump, or any change in the shape or feel of the breast, that may be an early sign of breast cancer.	All women, but especially those with a family history of breast cancer.	Examinations should start at puberty and be repeated every month at the same stage of the menstrual cycle.
TESTICLE EXAMINATION To detect any change in a testicle that may be an early sign of cancer.	All men.	Examinations should start at puberty and be repeated once a month, preferably after a warm bath or shower.

HEALTH CHECKUPS BY MEDICAL PROFESSIONALS

TEST AND PURPOSE	FOR WHOM RECOMMENDED	WHEN AND HOW OFTEN
CHILD DEVELOPMENT TESTS To monitor a child's growth and physical development and to detect any delay in the development of skills.	All children.	Begin at birth. Checkups are usually done at the ages of 2, 4, 6, 9, and 18 months, and then at 2 to 3 years, 5 to 6 years, and 10 to 11 years.
EYE EXAMINATION To detect any abnormality of vision or eye muscle disorder, and any sign of a general medical condition.	Anyone who has difficulty seeing, and anyone diagnosed as having diabetes or high blood pressure.	For those with eyesight problems, every 2 years. Those with good eyesight should begin at age 40 and retest every 2 years.
CERVICAL SMEAR (PAP TEST) To detect any abnormal cells in the cervix that might develop into cervical cancer.	All women who are currently sexually active or were sexually active in the past.	Begin soon after your first experience of sexual intercourse. Repeat 12 months later, and then at 1- to 3-year intervals for the rest of your life.
MEASUREMENT OF BLOOD PRESSURE To check the condition of the heart and arteries. High blood pressure may cause serious medical problems.	Anyone who has a family history of high blood pressure, heart or kidney disease, or stroke or diabetes, or who is overweight or taking the contraceptive pill.	Begin at the age of 20. Follow-ups should be every 3 to 5 years, or every year if you are taking the pill or are in a high-risk group.
BLOOD CHOLESTEROL TEST To detect people at high risk of coronary heart disease.	Anyone who has a family history of early-onset coronary heart disease.	Have the test done at the time of your periodic physical examination in your 20s.
MAMMOGRAPHY (BREAST X-RAY) To detect breast cancer before it becomes noticeable through physical examination.	Any woman who has a family history of breast cancer; all women over the age of 40.	Once between the ages of 35 and 40, every 1 to 2 years between the ages of 40 and 50; annually between ages 50 and 60.
RECTAL EXAMINATION To detect rectal cancer.	Anyone who has a family history of cancer of the colon or rectum in a close relative. All persons over the age of 50.	An annual digital rectal exam is advised after age 20. After age 50, stools should be tested for blood annually and a test with a proctosigmoidoscope should be conducted every 3 to 5 years.
DENTAL CHECKUP To examine the teeth, mouth, and gums for signs of decay, infection, or other problems.	Everyone. If you have not had regular checkups, start now rather than waiting until you have a problem.	Beginning in childhood, checkups should be carried out every 6 months before the age of 21, then every 1 to 2 years.
COMPLETE PHYSICAL EXAMINATION To check on the health of your heart, lungs, brain, and internal organs.	Anyone who has a family history of disorders of these organs and as a preventive measure for all others.	Once in your 20s, three times in your 30s, four times in your 40s, five times in your 50s, and annually thereafter.

pressure is persistently high (as is the case with one in four Americans), it puts your heart and blood vessels under greater strain. Untreated high blood pressure can cause a heart attack, heart failure, a stroke, or eye damage. Because high blood pressure causes no symptoms, it can be discovered only by regular tests by you or your doctor.

Testing the eyes

The ophthalmologist will test the sharpness of your vision by asking you to read the letters on a chart. You may then be prescribed glasses or contact lenses to correct any abnormality. The specialist may also perform a slit-lamp examination, using complex and powerful lenses to examine each part of your eye. A gauge may be rested in front of your eye to make sure the pressure in your eyeball is not abnormally high. You should have this measurement taken regularly, especially if anyone in your family has suffered from glaucoma.

Examining the retina
Your ophthalmologist may examine your eyes with an ophthalmoscope, an instrument that enables the structures at the back of the eye to be seen and any damage to the blood vessels in your retina to be detected.

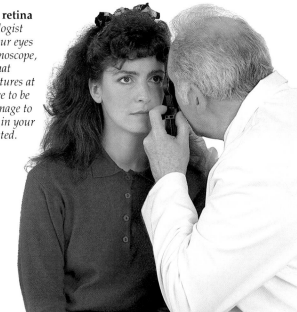

Dental care
A dental checkup involves much more than simply checking for tooth decay (below left). Your dentist will look for other problems affecting your teeth, gums, and mouth so that any treatment can be started early.

Checking child development

In the bustle of family life it is possible to overlook the fact that a child is not quite as responsive as others of his or her age. A child development examination is done to make sure that, should your child require treatment such as speech therapy or physical therapy, it can be implemented before the child has fallen too far behind others of the same age. Because hearing loss often goes unnoticed and can lead to further problems if untreated, the examination includes a test of your child's hearing.

CHILDHOOD IMMUNIZATION

Until the 1950s, most children suffered one or more of the serious infectious illnesses, such as diphtheria, measles, and pertussis (whooping cough). Many were very ill, a few died, but those who recovered never had that illness again. This natural ability of the body to "remember" each disease and defend itself against it is called acquired immunity.

Immunization tricks the body into mounting its defenses against a mild form of a disease, thus preparing it to fight off a genuine attack. The immuni-

Mouth lining
Checked for any abnormality.

Biting surfaces
Checked for decay, chipping, staining, and erosion.

Gums
Checked for inflammation, swelling, and bleeding.

Other tooth surfaces
Checked for plaque and calculus.

Tooth relationships
Checked for bite, crowding, and signs of irregular wear.

zation program has been so successful that parents can overlook the fact that infectious diseases can still be serious and life threatening. By having your child immunized, you protect him or her against diphtheria, polio, tetanus, measles, mumps, rubella, and pertussis.

How is immunization done?

Although there are very few reasons a child should not receive a specific immunization, you should always check with your doctor beforehand. Once an examination is made, immunization may be performed at a special center or in the doctor's office. It generally involves an injection into the upper arm or the buttock, either into a muscle or into the tissues under the skin. Polio vaccine is taken by mouth, usually on a sugar cube.

What are the aftereffects?

Immunization usually carries no aftereffects. Your child should remain at the health facility or doctor's office for at least 10 minutes in case there is any immediate allergic reaction. If he or she vomits within 30 minutes of swallowing the polio vaccine, another dose of the vaccine will need to be given.

Occasionally, pain, tenderness, and swelling develop around the injection site. Children may become feverish and suffer influenzalike symptoms for a day

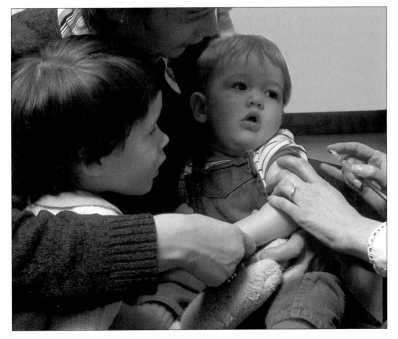

or two, may cry more than usual, become irritable, or stop eating. Acetaminophen should be given to any child who has a fever. Some vaccines cause a mild form of the disease. A rash develops in some children a few days after they receive the measles immunization, but they are not infectious to anyone in contact with them.

A severe reaction to immunization is extremely rare. If a child starts to scream or cry continuously, becomes drowsy or restless, vomits several times, has difficulty breathing, has swelling of the face or lips, or has a seizure, call your doctor.

Receiving a vaccine
Most toddlers tolerate vaccination with no more than minor distress.

Is whooping cough vaccine dangerous?

You may have read or heard about children suffering brain damage after receiving the pertussis (whooping cough) vaccine. The risk of brain damage is small – less than one in 100,000. There is a much greater risk of serious illness, handicap, or death from having pertussis than from a reaction to the vaccine. Several years ago in the United Kingdom, concern about the pertussis vaccination led to many children not being immunized. A subsequent epidemic of pertussis caused the deaths of 30 children.

CHILDHOOD IMMUNIZATION SCHEDULE			
To protect your child early in life, he or she should be immunized at the ages shown.	AGE	COMBINED INJECTION	ORAL
	2 months	Diphtheria, pertussis (whooping cough), tetanus	Poliomyelitis·
	4 months	Diphtheria, pertussis, tetanus	Poliomyelitis
	6 months	Diphtheria, pertussis, tetanus	
	15 months	Measles, mumps, rubella (German measles)	
	18 months	Diphtheria, pertussis, tetanus	Poliomyelitis
	4 to 6 years	Diphtheria, pertussis, tetanus	Poliomyelitis

CHAPTER TWO

MANAGING COMMON HEALTH PROBLEMS

DOCTORS SOMETIMES say that one third of patients wait too long before asking for help, one third ask too soon, and only the remaining third judge correctly when to seek assistance. This chapter is designed to help you understand the nature of most common health problems and to decide when to call your doctor, or when to wait and see whether your symptoms improve or get worse. Real medical emergencies – a sudden collapse with loss of consciousness, vomiting blood, loss of vision, or a severe, unremitting pain in the abdomen – are uncommon and dramatic. Other reasons for immediate medical concern may be less obvious, so you need to know the main patterns of illness that should prompt you to ask for help *immediately*. By contrast, each of us has experienced common symptoms, such as a headache, diarrhea, back pain,

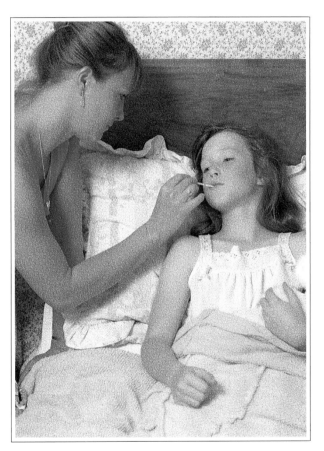

or a sore throat, that have cleared up without treatment within 24 to 48 hours. Asking for medical advice about such symptoms in the first few hours is usually unnecessary. What you *can* do is to follow some simple self-help measures to relieve discomfort and, possibly, reduce the risk of progression to a more serious disorder. Much of this chapter is divided into the anatomical areas where common symp-

toms occur – for example, the upper respiratory tract (the site of coughs and colds), chest, back, digestive system, skin, eyes, and ears. In addition, vague feelings of "feeling under the weather," abnormal behavior, and special problems of children are covered in sections of their own. The information is presented in several different ways. The MONITOR YOUR SYMPTOMS charts will guide you to possible causes of symptoms and the actions required. Along with the HELPLINE diagrams, these guides will alert you to the circumstances in which a doctor should be called without delay. The ASK YOUR DOCTOR columns provide answers to some of the common questions posed about health and medicine – perhaps questions you may have forgotten or been too embarrassed to ask the last time you paid a visit to your doctor. Although taking charge of your health is a theme of this chapter, the objective is not to discourage you from seeking medical help. The CASE HISTORY features illustrate your doctor's skills in recognizing disorders quickly and accurately. No two illnesses are ever exactly the same. However, you may find similarities to your own medical problems in these case histories, and thus gain insight into the nature of an illness through the experiences of others.

AN ILLNESS IN THE FAMILY

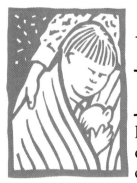

K NOWING THE BEST course of action to take when a member of your family feels sick is not always easy. Common symptoms, such as a sore throat, a headache, or diarrhea, may clear up within 48 hours of their own accord. In other cases, they may be an indication of a more serious illness. Whatever the outcome, it is worthwhile to chart the course of any illness so that you can give your doctor a detailed account of how it has progressed.

The initial assessment
When a member of the family complains of feeling sick, be alert to a few basic signs. Feeling the forehead for raised temperature or checking the complexion for pallor and the chest for any rash should be part of the initial assessment.

When the symptoms of illness first appear, it is not usually possible for anyone, even the most skilled doctor, to forecast with accuracy how long the illness will last or how severe it will be. A headache, for example, may be the first symptom of a prolonged attack of influenza, or it may disappear within a few hours. An attack of nasal stuffiness may or may not progress to acute bronchitis. As a general rule, however, there is cause for concern only when the person's condition becomes worse rather than better within the first 48 hours.

MONITORING SYMPTOMS AND SIGNS

In medical terms, symptoms are the features of an illness that are obvious to the sufferer but not to anyone else. All forms of pain fit into this category – only the sufferer knows how bad the pain is, when it has begun to get better, and when it has cleared up completely. Thus, the first task in managing an illness is to gain a clear picture of the symptoms, and to update that picture every few hours to establish whether the symptoms are worsening or improving.

Checking appearance
In contrast to symptoms, the aspects of health problems that can be seen or measured by others are known medically as "signs." Someone who feels ill may also look ill. He or she may be pale, may be sweating, or may be breathing more rapidly than usual. Thus, the second task in managing an illness is to check on the sick family member's outward appearance and behavior. There may be a rash or swelling on part of the body, one of the person's eyes may be red, or the person may be using the toilet more often than usual. Make a note of these and any other significant changes (see CHARTING THE COURSE OF AN ILLNESS, page 32). Your doctor may ask you to record basic signs such as pulse and temperature, especially in the case of a sick child.

Taking the temperature

Using a thermometer to monitor temperature is the third task in managing an illness. Normal body temperature is about 98.6°F (37°C) but may vary by about 1 to 2°F (0.5 to 1°C) throughout the day. A higher than normal temperature (a fever) in a previously healthy person is not in itself dangerous unless it exceeds 104°F (40°C). Beyond this point, the body's temperature-control system begins to become ineffective.

The temperature should be taken about once every 4 hours and any change noted. A rise in temperature is usually caused either by infection or injury.

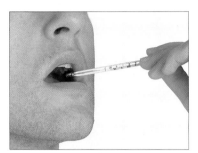

1 Holding the thermometer at the opposite end from the bulb, shake it down to drive the mercury level well below the normal mark.

2 Slide the thermometer under the patient's tongue and ask him or her to close the mouth. The thermometer can also be placed under an armpit.

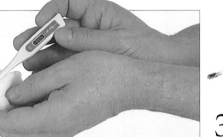

Digital thermometer
A digital thermometer gives a quicker temperature measurement than a mercury thermometer and is easier to read. However, it is less accurate.

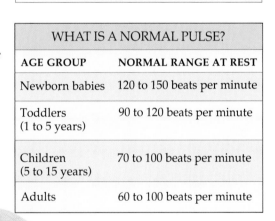

Reading

3 After 3 minutes, remove the thermometer and read the top of the mercury column against the scale.

Measuring the pulse
Locate the pulse with two fingers placed on the palm side of the wrist below the base of the thumb. Count the number of beats over a full minute (or over 30 seconds and multiply the number by two).

WHAT IS A NORMAL PULSE?	
AGE GROUP	**NORMAL RANGE AT REST**
Newborn babies	120 to 150 beats per minute
Toddlers (1 to 5 years)	90 to 120 beats per minute
Children (5 to 15 years)	70 to 100 beats per minute
Adults	60 to 100 beats per minute

Taking the pulse

Measuring the pulse may help your doctor in the assessment and management of an illness. With each heartbeat you can feel a pulse throb wherever a large artery lies near the skin's surface. One method of taking the pulse (and the range of normal resting pulse rates) is shown at left. During sleep the pulse rate falls by 10 to 20 beats per minute.

Infection, shock, and heart disease are among the possible causes of a raised heart rate, but the rate also rises during exercise, so the pulse should be taken with the patient relaxed. Hypothermia (a dangerous drop below normal in body temperature) can cause the heart to beat more slowly than usual. If you measure a pulse outside the normal range, or note any significant change in a person's pulse during an illness, report it to your doctor. It is wise to keep a record of the normal pulse rates of all family members as a basis for comparison.

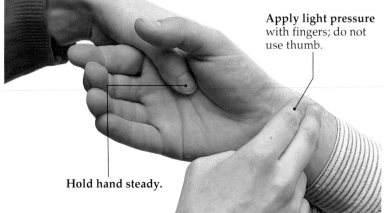

Apply light pressure with fingers; do not use thumb.

Hold hand steady.

RECORDING FAMILY ILLNESSES

Keeping a written diary of the course of an illness fulfills several useful functions. First, keeping track of the temperature and pulse gives an objective guide to whether the illness is getting better or worse. Second, a record of these signs will help if you need to consult your doctor and will assist him or her in making a diagnosis. Third, the diary can be used to remind you of when medications were last given – and when they need to be given next. You can also record any special instructions for administering the medication.

In addition to providing a record of temperature, pulse, and medications, the diary will help you remember how the sick person felt from time to time, occurrences such as vomiting or diarrhea, the level of fluid and food intake, the frequency of sleep, and anything else you feel might be significant.

CHARTING THE COURSE OF AN ILLNESS

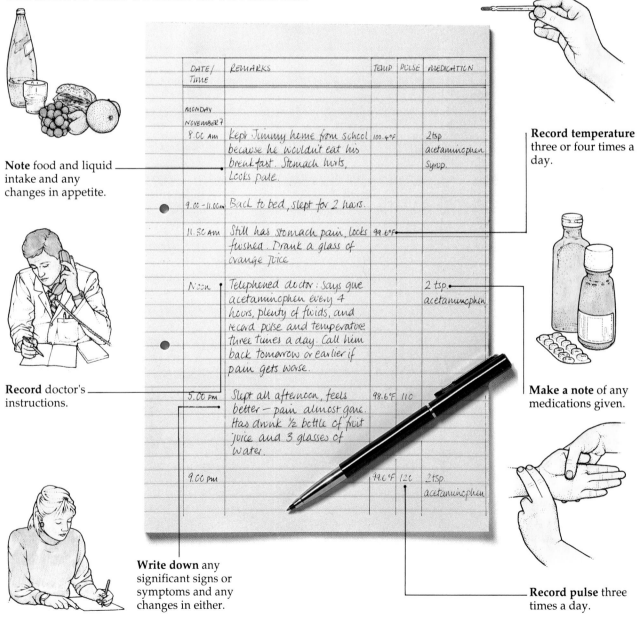

Note food and liquid intake and any changes in appetite.

Record doctor's instructions.

Write down any significant signs or symptoms and any changes in either.

Record temperature three or four times a day.

Make a note of any medications given.

Record pulse three times a day.

HELPLINE
SUDDEN ILLNESS

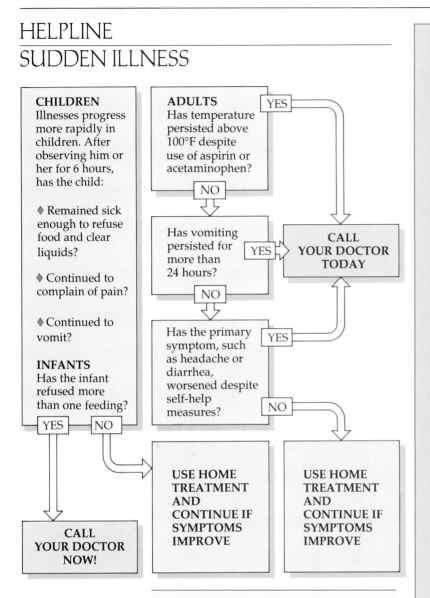

CHILDREN
Illnesses progress more rapidly in children. After observing him or her for 6 hours, has the child:

♦ Remained sick enough to refuse food and clear liquids?

♦ Continued to complain of pain?

♦ Continued to vomit?

INFANTS
Has the infant refused more than one feeding?

YES   NO

ADULTS
Has temperature persisted above 100°F despite use of aspirin or acetaminophen?

YES

NO

Has vomiting persisted for more than 24 hours?

YES

NO

Has the primary symptom, such as headache or diarrhea, worsened despite self-help measures?

YES

NO

CALL YOUR DOCTOR TODAY

CALL YOUR DOCTOR NOW!

USE HOME TREATMENT AND CONTINUE IF SYMPTOMS IMPROVE

USE HOME TREATMENT AND CONTINUE IF SYMPTOMS IMPROVE

MANAGING THE ILLNESS

If you or someone in your family has a single complaint, such as a sore throat, it makes little sense to attempt a diagnosis of the underlying cause. Provided there are no serious grounds for concern (see WARNING box at right), the best course of action is simply to use self-help measures to treat the symptom at home. However, it is important to monitor the symptoms carefully and reassess the situation regularly over a period of 48 hours. If there is no improvement during this time, if any new symptoms develop, or if the original symptoms get worse, you should call your doctor.

WARNING

Most common medical symptoms can be treated safely at home for an initial 48 hours, but there are some circumstances in which you should call your doctor or an ambulance immediately.

♦ **Unexplained drowsiness or loss of consciousness.** If someone becomes sleepy and cannot be brought back to full alertness, there are grounds for concern. Possible causes may include an overdose of drugs, a brain disorder such as meningitis, or a biochemical upset such as uncontrolled diabetes.

♦ **Severe bleeding.** The patient's life may be threatened if blood spurts from a wound (suggesting artery damage), if more than half a pint of blood is lost, or if first-aid measures fail to stop the bleeding within 5 minutes.

♦ **Crushing central chest pain that is not relieved by rest.** This symptom may be due to a heart attack, especially if accompanied by weakness, pallor, sweating, and a pain in the arm.

♦ **Shortness of breath or difficulty breathing** (wheezing) in anyone sitting down or lying down in bed. Anyone with asthma or bronchitis who does not respond to his or her usual treatment may also require immediate help; these are potentially life-threatening conditions.

♦ **Severe abdominal pain** that is not relieved by vomiting or if accompanied by sweating or faintness, or any abdominal pain localized to one side of the abdomen that persists for more than 3 hours. These types of abdominal pain should be investigated immediately; the cause may be a serious problem such as appendicitis.

♦ **Blurred vision** that has developed rapidly. It can have many possible serious causes, including glaucoma.

HOME MEDICINE CABINET

Here is a collection of items that are useful to have in your home medicine cabinet. Other items may be required according to your individual needs.

STORING DRUGS
♦ Store drugs in the containers in which they were originally purchased.
♦ Replace caps and lids securely after use.

THROW AWAY
♦ Any prescribed drugs you are not taking.
♦ Any tablets or capsules that are discolored, disintegrating, softened, stuck together, or that smell different from the original.
♦ Any tablets or capsules that are more than 2 years old. Liquids that smell or taste different from the original or are thickened or discolored.
♦ Tubes that are hard, cracked, or leaky, and any ointments or creams that have changed their odor or have hardened or discolored.

SKIN CONDITIONS

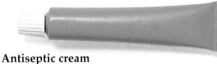

Antiseptic cream
Containing an antiseptic for preventing infection in minor cuts and scrapes.

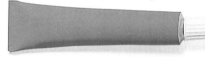

Antifungal cream
Containing an antifungus medication for athlete's foot, "jock itch," and other fungal skin infections.

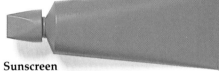

Sunscreen
Always apply before sun exposure.

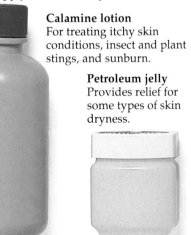

Calamine lotion
For treating itchy skin conditions, insect and plant stings, and sunburn.

Petroleum jelly
Provides relief for some types of skin dryness.

PRESCRIBED DRUGS
Should be used only by the person for whom they have been prescribed.

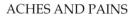

ACHES AND PAINS

Aspirin tablets
Relieve all types of pain and reduce fever. For use by adults over age 16.

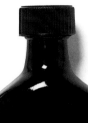

Liniment
Liquid containing methyl salicylate for relief of muscle aches and pains.

Acetaminophen tablets
Relieve pain and reduce fever. Suitable for children and adults.

Acetaminophen syrup
More acceptable than tablets to children.

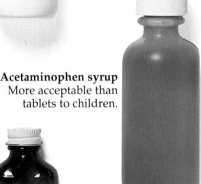

Oil of cloves
Useful temporary relief for toothache.

GENERAL EQUIPMENT

Thermometer
Use for taking the temperature.

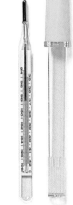

Eye cup
Use with water to float off foreign particles in the eye.

Cotton swabs
For delicate cleansing (but not for use in the ear canal).

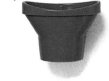

DIGESTIVE TRACT
PROBLEMS AND
EMERGENCIES

Ipecac
Induces vomiting of
swallowed, non-
corrosive, poisonous
material in an
emergency. Always
call a hospital
emergency room or a
poison control center
before use.

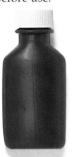

Antacid mixture
Containing a calcium or
aluminum/magnesium
antacid to relieve heartburn
and indigestion.

Rehydration powders
Added to water, are used to
prevent or treat dehydration
caused by severe diarrhea or
vomiting.

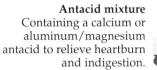

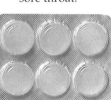

Antidiarrhea medication
Containing an antidiarrheal for treatment of diarrhea. Do not give to children
or use without consulting a doctor if you have a fever for more
than 48 hours.

MOUTH, NOSE, AND
THROAT

Antiseptic mouthwash
For sore mouth or mouth
ulceration.

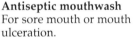

Antihistamine tablets
For relief of allergic nasal
stuffiness or hay fever.

Throat lozenges
Useful for easing
the pain of a
sore throat.

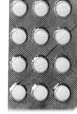

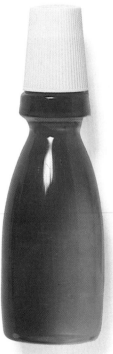

Cough expectorant
Loosens phlegm, allowing it
to be more easily coughed up.
Do not use cough remedies
for more than 48 hours
without consulting a doctor.

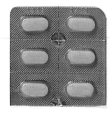

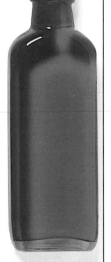

Decongestant tablets
Help to reduce nasal stuffiness caused by colds or flu.

In many cases, the symptoms clear up
before you seek medical help. For example, a 24-hour diet of no solid food
and plenty of clear fluids usually ends a
bout of diarrhea. Many cases of headache and back pain resolve themselves
while you rest quietly in bed.

Medications

For certain symptoms, over-the-counter
medications can be useful (see opposite). Painkillers such as aspirin for adults
or acetaminophen for children and teenagers under age 16 will relieve the pain
of a sore throat and make swallowing
easier. Painkillers can also be used to
bring down a temperature and may help
relieve headaches. Symptoms such as
these can be treated by anyone, without
risk, during the first 48 hours in which
the symptoms are present.

Certain precautions should be taken
with any medication, however. Always
read the directions on the label and follow them carefully. Do not continue use
of the medication for a prolonged period
without consulting your doctor, and
always stop the medication if you notice
any unpleasant or alarming side effects.
Also avoid using several different
medications at the same time to treat a
single symptom.

Antibiotics

One group of medications that should
definitely not be used to treat common
conditions, except under the direction
of a doctor, are antibiotics.

There are several reasons for this. First,
self-treatment with antibiotics may
change your symptoms in such a way
that the underlying illness becomes less
easy to identify. Second, like all powerful drugs, antibiotics can have unpleasant side effects, which may be worse
than the original symptom. Third, antibiotics are effective only against certain
types of infection, mainly those caused
by bacteria. They are completely ineffective against noninfectious illnesses and
against infections such as influenza and
colds, which are caused by viruses.

FEELING UNDER THE WEATHER

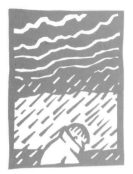

W E ALL HAVE DAYS when we feel out of sorts. The symptoms of feeling under the weather may include tiredness, lack of energy, weakness, and an aching body. The causes of these symptoms are numerous. In general, anyone who feels sick for more than a few days should consult a doctor to make sure that there is no serious underlying disorder.

Fatigue and lethargy
Vague feelings of tiredness may have causes ranging from overuse of alcohol and caffeine to hormonal upsets or the onset of an infectious illness.

When a person complains of feeling under the weather, it usually means that he or she has a variety of vague symptoms that are unrelated to any specific serious illness. There are many possible causes for these symptoms, including the early stages of an infection such as influenza. Our life-style can also undermine good health, and problems such as anxiety or depression may be accompanied by physical effects. Hormonal conditions such as hypothyroidism (a disorder of the thyroid gland) may bring on tiredness and weakness. The onset of the menopause causes some hormonal readjustments, which affect women in different ways. Some women feel unusually tired and depressed during this period of their lives. Finally, feeling generally "off " may be the first indication of a more serious underlying medical problem.

EARLY WARNINGS OF ILLNESS

A general "run-down" feeling is a common early sign that a more specific disorder may be on the way. Viral illnesses such as influenza or the common cold often start with an overall aching and weariness. Doctors sometimes call such symptoms the "prodrome," or forerunner, of the illness. More specific symptoms, such as a sore throat, a runny nose, or a high temperature, appear only later. The same sense of debilitation can also persist for several days after the other symptoms have cleared up.

The early stages of severe anemia, rheumatic diseases such as rheumatoid arthritis and lupus erythematosus, and all types of cancer can cause you to feel sick. In most of these cases, however, other symptoms would prompt you to make an appointment with your doctor.

Prolonged periods of fatigue

Illnesses such as glandular fever can cause tiredness and lethargy for many months after other symptoms are gone. If you are one of the few who suffer from a prolonged, run-down feeling, your doctor may say you are suffering from postviral

COULD SMOKING, ALCOHOL, OR CAFFEINE BE TO BLAME?

Though they are tolerated socially to varying degrees, alcohol, caffeine, and tobacco are all drugs. Many people use them initially for the short-term pleasant feelings they give. In heavy users, however, the primary reason for continued use may be to avoid unpleasant with-drawal symptoms. Occasional overuse of any of these substances can make you feel run-down and sluggish; regular overuse of any of these addictive drugs is virtually a prescription for illness and serious damage to your health.

EFFECTS OF CAFFEINE

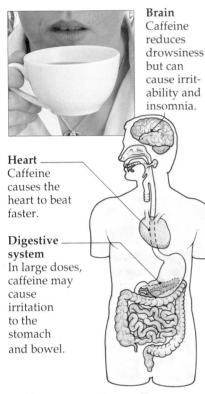

Brain
Caffeine reduces drowsiness but can cause irritability and insomnia.

Heart
Caffeine causes the heart to beat faster.

Digestive system
In large doses, caffeine may cause irritation to the stomach and bowel.

Caffeine-containing coffee, tea, and colas carry variable amounts of this stimulant substance. If you drink five or more cups of strong coffee, or 12 or more cups of tea a day, you are probably taking in more than half a gram of caffeine – a large quantity of a relatively powerful drug.

Caffeine affects many parts of the body. In addition to those shown above, it stimulates the kidneys to produce more urine. Large doses can cause restlessness in the evening and may leave you feeling drowsy the next morning. Overstimulation of the heart muscle can cause palpitations, and irritation of the digestive system makes any stomach ulcer worse. If you have any of these symptoms, it may be worth trying a caffeine-free day.

THE ALCOHOLIC HANGOVER

The short-term effects of excess alcohol consumption are best illustrated by the hangover – the combination of headache, nausea, vomiting, vertigo, and thirst experienced by the drinker the morning after heavy drinking.

Some of the main symptoms of a hangover are explained below. The headache may be caused by alcohol itself, by its breakdown products, or by congeners (secondary products of alcohol fermentation, present in drinks such as bourbon and red wine). A hangover is often made worse by carbon monoxide absorbed from cigarette smoke.

Although small amounts of alcohol have less drastic effects, it is a good idea to keep a few days each week alcohol-free.

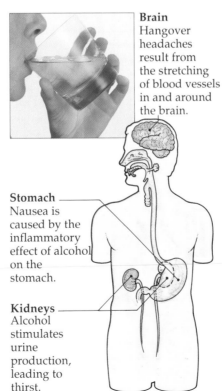

Brain
Hangover headaches result from the stretching of blood vessels in and around the brain.

Stomach
Nausea is caused by the inflammatory effect of alcohol on the stomach.

Kidneys
Alcohol stimulates urine production, leading to thirst.

EFFECTS OF SMOKING

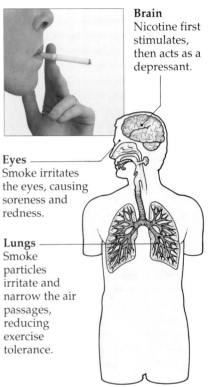

Brain
Nicotine first stimulates, then acts as a depressant.

Eyes
Smoke irritates the eyes, causing soreness and redness.

Lungs
Smoke particles irritate and narrow the air passages, reducing exercise tolerance.

The long-term ill effects of smoking on health have been well publicized. Less clear, perhaps, are the unpleasant short- to medium-term effects that smoking also can have.

In addition to the effects shown above, smoke particles cause inflammation and increased mucus production in the lining of the lung airways. This condition leads to a smoker's cough (a general term to describe chronic bronchitis) and, from time to time, chest pain.

Smoking also leaves the mouth feeling dry and stale and causes the breath to have an offensive odor. Like alcohol and caffeine, smoking can aggravate a peptic ulcer.

If you are a smoker, try to quit now; you'll live longer and feel better once you have given up the habit.

MONITOR YOUR SYMPTOMS
FATIGUE AND LETHARGY

All of us occasionally feel unusually tired and lethargic, even though there may be no specific reason for it. Minor infections are a common cause; the condition may also be the result of an unhealthy life-style. If fatigue and lethargy persist, they may be signs of a more serious disorder that requires your doctor's attention.

BEGIN HERE

Do you often feel ill at ease, or do you experience periods of low spirits accompanied by indecisiveness, a loss of appetite, loss of energy, or a lack of interest in sex?

YES

NO

The action of certain drugs may make you feel dull and sluggish.
Are you taking any medications?

YES

NO

Action If you suspect your medication is having the side effect of making you feel tired, discuss this possibility with your doctor.

NO

NO

You may be suffering from anxiety or depression:

Anxiety A common cause of anxiety is excessive stress at work or at home. You may be tense and apprehensive, find it difficult to concentrate, be short-tempered with family and colleagues, and sleep poorly.

Action If your anxiety persists after a reduction in the stresses in your life, see your doctor.

Depression Persistent low spirits, often accompanied by feelings of futility and guilt, may be caused by too much stress or by an unhappy event such as bereavement or divorce. Some people regularly feel depressed despite the absence of any obvious outside cause.

Action Your doctor may be able to suggest some techniques to combat your depression. If your depression is severe, he or she may prescribe a short-term medication to help you out of the depressive episode.

Feelings of lethargy often accompany a fever.
Do you have a temperature of 100°F (38°C) or above?

YES

Fever (abnormally high body temperature) is most often a sign that your body is fighting infection. A viral infection is a strong possibility. Infections may also cause depression and tiredness during the recovery period, which can last for several weeks.

Action Consult your doctor if your temperature remains raised for longer than 48 hours, or rises above 104°F (40°C). During convalescence, make sure you eat a nourishing diet and rest until you feel well again.

Feeling worn out during the day may be the result of insufficient or disturbed sleep.
Are you having problems with getting enough sleep at night?

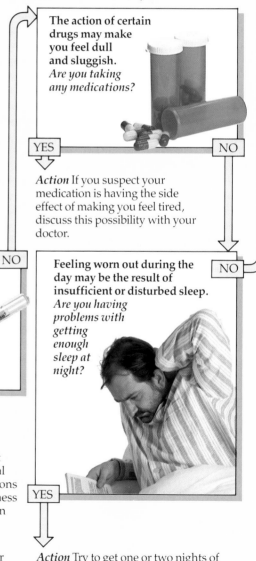

YES

YES

Action Try to get one or two nights of sound, unbroken sleep. Consult your doctor if you find it difficult to get to sleep, or if you keep waking up during the night.

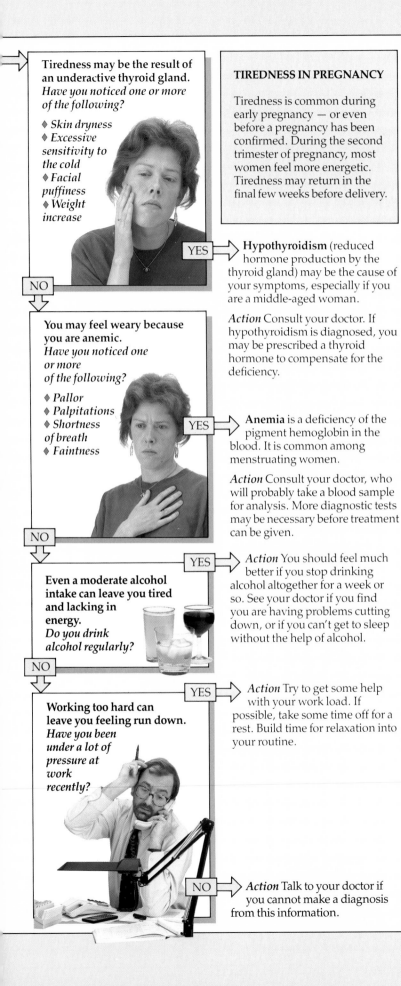

Tiredness may be the result of an underactive thyroid gland. *Have you noticed one or more of the following?*

♦ *Skin dryness*
♦ *Excessive sensitivity to the cold*
♦ *Facial puffiness*
♦ *Weight increase*

YES

NO

TIREDNESS IN PREGNANCY

Tiredness is common during early pregnancy — or even before a pregnancy has been confirmed. During the second trimester of pregnancy, most women feel more energetic. Tiredness may return in the final few weeks before delivery.

Hypothyroidism (reduced hormone production by the thyroid gland) may be the cause of your symptoms, especially if you are a middle-aged woman.

Action Consult your doctor. If hypothyroidism is diagnosed, you may be prescribed a thyroid hormone to compensate for the deficiency.

You may feel weary because you are anemic. *Have you noticed one or more of the following?*

♦ *Pallor*
♦ *Palpitations*
♦ *Shortness of breath*
♦ *Faintness*

YES

NO

Anemia is a deficiency of the pigment hemoglobin in the blood. It is common among menstruating women.

Action Consult your doctor, who will probably take a blood sample for analysis. More diagnostic tests may be necessary before treatment can be given.

Even a moderate alcohol intake can leave you tired and lacking in energy. *Do you drink alcohol regularly?*

YES

NO

Action You should feel much better if you stop drinking alcohol altogether for a week or so. See your doctor if you find you are having problems cutting down, or if you can't get to sleep without the help of alcohol.

Working too hard can leave you feeling run down. *Have you been under a lot of pressure at work recently?*

YES

NO

Action Try to get some help with your work load. If possible, take some time off for a rest. Build time for relaxation into your routine.

Action Talk to your doctor if you cannot make a diagnosis from this information.

fatigue syndrome. Not every doctor accepts this diagnosis, however, and some specialists attribute the symptoms to tension and strain rather than the aftermath of a viral illness. Most people recover with time, helped by getting enough rest and trying to identify and deal with causes of emotional stress.

Anxiety and depression

You may feel sick because you are unhappy at work or at home. Anxiety can cause symptoms of nervous tension such as a dry mouth, difficulty swallowing, tremor, diarrhea, and a sensation of butterflies in the stomach. Depression often results in constipation, loss of appetite, reduced sex drive, and difficulty concentrating. All of these symptoms improve when the anxiety or depression is resolved.

Apart from causing this evidence that your body is under duress, anxiety and depression undermine your health by interrupting your sleep. In addition, they can make it difficult for you to fall asleep, may cause you to sleep excessively, or may cause you to wake up in the early hours of the morning. Remember that regular sleep patterns are an invaluable aid to good health. It is particularly important that the cause of any developing pattern of excessive or deficient sleep be addressed and corrected before your health is affected by it.

HORMONAL DISORDERS

Tiredness and lethargy may be caused by a hormonal disorder such as hypothyroidism or diabetes. These disorders are also accompanied by specific symptoms. Hypothyroidism usually brings weight gain, dry skin, brittle hair, puffiness of the face, and excessive sensitivity to the cold. The presence of a hormonal disorder can be confirmed by your doctor by analysis of a blood sample.

Premenstrual syndrome

Premenstrual syndrome (PMS) may cause a woman to feel different from her

39

usual self in the days just before her menstrual period each month. She may feel lethargic, bloated, tense, and irritable, as well as more clumsy than usual. PMS is thought to be caused by a disorder in the body's regulation of hormone balance. Possible causes include a fall in the production of the hormone progesterone, a deficiency of the hormone estrogen, or a disorder in the way the chemicals in the central nervous system (brain and spinal cord) interact with progesterone and estrogen.

The menopause

Tiredness often accompanies the menopause. In women whose periods get heavier before they cease, the tiredness may be caused by anemia. Other symptoms may include hot flashes, night sweats, headaches, and palpitations. However, some women go through this phase of their lives with few symptoms, or none at all.

DRUG SIDE EFFECTS

Some prescription drugs, including decongestants, tranquilizers, beta-blockers, appetite suppressants and bronchodilators, may make you feel tired and lethargic because they disrupt the quality of your sleep. Other drugs affect the way you feel for different reasons. Diuretics can lower the potassium level in your body, antibiotics can slow the production of cell proteins, and anticonvulsants suppress nerve activity in your brain. If your medication is making you feel sick, inform your doctor.

HOW TO BEAT INSOMNIA

Tiredness, lethargy, and a general feeling of being run-down are often the result of sleep loss. People vary a great deal in the amount of sleep they need, but no matter how many hours you like to sleep, it is important that you wake up feeling rested and refreshed. If you have difficulty getting to sleep, or lie awake for long periods in the middle of the night, some of these suggestions may help you achieve a more satisfying sleep pattern.

Rest and relaxation
♦ Try to do some form of physical exercise during the day, preferably in the fresh air, so that you feel tired at bedtime.
♦ Allow yourself at least 1 hour of relaxation before bed, especially if you work late or feel stressed and tense at the end of a busy day. A warm bath before going to bed may help.
♦ Avoid taking naps during the day. They will only make the problem worse.

Eating and drinking
♦ Do not eat your main evening meal too late; an active digestive system inhibits sleep. You should allow at least 2 hours between eating and going to bed.
♦ Avoid drinking stimulants, such as coffee and tea, or large amounts of alcohol before bed. A warm milky drink will promote sleep by helping you relax.

Anxiety and stress
♦ Worries about work, money, and personal relationships are perhaps the principal cause of long periods of wakefulness during the night. You can attempt to reduce your feelings of anxiety by focusing your mind on a less stressful subject, such as an upcoming vacation or a favorite leisure activity.
♦ If your worries get the better of you, get up and occupy yourself with an activity that will take your mind off your problems.
♦ Do not use sleeping pills, except under the supervision of your doctor.

Peace and quiet
♦ Sleep on a firm, comfortable mattress.
♦ Make sure that your bedroom is neither too hot nor too cold.
♦ If light in the bedroom or background noise disturbs your sleep, you may find that an eye shade and earplugs will help you block out these distractions.

CASE HISTORY
FATIGUE AND WEIGHT GAIN

JOAN HAD NOT been feeling well for several weeks. She felt extremely tired most of the time and was finding it difficult to concentrate on her work at the bank. She was also depressed about her appearance because, despite regular exercise and following a strict diet, her weight had increased considerably in the last 2 months.

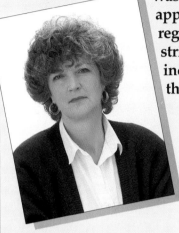

PERSONAL DETAILS
Name Joan Thompson
Age 52
Occupation Bank teller
Family Father is in good health, apart from arthritis in his knees. Mother suffers from pernicious anemia.

MEDICAL BACKGROUND
Joan had her tonsils and adenoids taken out as a child, and her appendix was removed at the age of 14. Apart from regular Pap smears done by her gynecologist, she has not seen a doctor for many years.

THE CONSULTATION
Joan asks her doctor for something to help her lose weight. She tells him that, despite her efforts to prevent it, she has put on almost 22 pounds over the last few months. Joan is worried because she begins to feel tired and sleepy within 2 hours of waking up in the morning. In addition, she has been feeling cold and has been suffering from constipation for several months.

During the physical examination, the doctor checks her pulse and detects a slow heart rate of 50 beats per minute. Her blood pressure is normal and there is no sign of anemia. He then carefully examines her thyroid gland and finds it enlarged, causing a smooth swelling across the front of her neck.

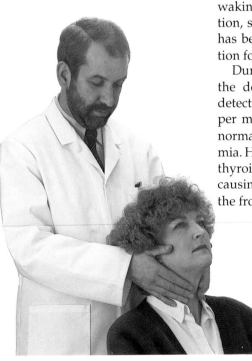

Examining the thyroid gland
If the thyroid is under-active, hormonal control systems cause some compensatory enlargement of the gland, which can be felt by the doctor during an examination.

THE DOCTOR'S IMPRESSION
Joan's symptoms point to hypothyroidism – her thyroid gland is underactive and is not producing sufficient thyroid hormones. Cells throughout her body are not receiving the hormones they need and, because the function of thyroid hormones is to stimulate chemical reactions in the cells, many of her body's normal activities have slowed down. This accounts for her feelings of fatigue and cold; her cells are not producing enough energy. Similar factors have caused her digestive system to slow down, causing constipation, and her heart rate to drop. Because the calories in her food are not being used up at a normal rate, Joan has gained weight.

Joan's doctor tests a blood sample and, as he expects, low levels of thyroid hormones are found.

THE DIAGNOSIS
The most common cause of hypothyroidism is an autoimmune disease, in which the body's defense system destroys cells in the thyroid gland. Joan's blood sample indicates a raised level of antibodies against thyroid cells, confirming her doctor's diagnosis of AUTOIMMUNE HYPOTHYROIDISM.

THE TREATMENT
Joan is given a low dose of synthetic thyroid hormone to supplement her deficiency. Within a month she is feeling more energetic and she is not as tired. Slowly the dose of hormones is increased until, after 6 months, the correct amount for her is established. By then, her weight has returned to normal. She will need to continue the synthetic hormone treatment daily for the rest of her life. A checkup and blood test will be required annually, but her health is now good.

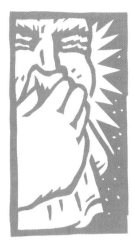

COUGHS, COLDS, AND INFLUENZA

A SORE THROAT, RUNNY NOSE, hacking cough, chills – we are all acquainted with the miseries of colds and flu. However, despite years of research, a cure for these common ailments is as elusive as ever, and today they continue to account for almost one quarter of all consultations with family doctors.

The upper respiratory tract is continuously exposed to potentially infectious microorganisms such as viruses and bacteria. Although the body's immune system fights any such invading organisms, respiratory infections caused by a viral attack are almost impossible to avoid because there are so many different types of viruses. Depending on the type of virus we catch and the areas it infects, a variety of illnesses may result.

THE COMMON COLD

The common cold, or "head" cold, is a minor infectious illness that affects the nose, throat, and sinuses. It can be caused by any one of nearly 200 different viruses. Exact symptoms may vary from virus to virus, but a typical cold manifests itself in a blocked or runny nose,

Viral infection
An electron micrograph image of cold viruses surrounding a host body cell is shown below. The viruses appear as small pink dots around the wall of the larger orange cell; the bright red forms are red blood cells. After the initial infection of the upper respiratory tract, cold viruses multiply and spread extremely rapidly.

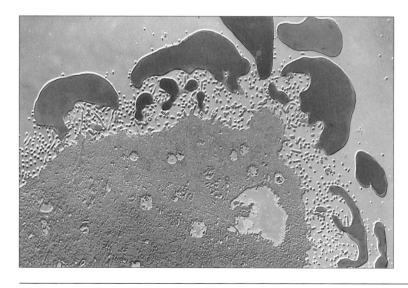

watery eyes, sneezing, sore throat, coughing, and hoarseness. In addition, you may suffer a slight fever and feelings of tiredness. These symptoms usually clear up in 3 or 4 days, although the nasal symptoms may persist.

Can colds be avoided?

Everybody catches colds, but children and young adults acquire them more frequently than older people because their bodies have not yet built up immunity. They are thus vulnerable to a wider range of cold viruses. As you grow older, your body acquires extra immunity to cold viruses with every cold you catch, so you become less susceptible to infection. There is no certain method of avoiding colds. There is also no evidence to support the idea that vitamin C or other vitamin supplements help ward off infection, or that colds are brought on by drafty environments or by getting soaked in the cold rain.

What is the treatment?

There is no cure or effective preventive measure for the common cold. You can ease the symptoms by staying warm, drinking plenty of fluids, and by taking aspirin (children under the age of 16 should *not* take aspirin) or acetaminophen. Over-the-counter cold remedies used in moderation may also provide some temporary relief. However, if your symptoms persist for more than 7 days, consult your doctor.

INFECTIONS OF THE UPPER AIRWAYS

Viral and bacterial infections can affect different areas of the upper respiratory tract, producing a range of illnesses generally called the common cold. These illnesses are in fact separate disorders, but a cold sufferer is usually affected by several of them at once.

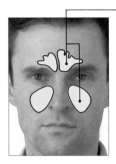

Sinusitis
Inflammation of the mucous membranes lining the sinus cavities. Symptoms include a headache above the eyes and painful cheeks.

Nasal infection
Infection of the mucous membranes of the nasal passage, causing sneezing and a stuffy or runny nose.

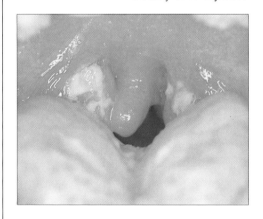

Tonsillitis
Acute inflammation of the tonsils, situated on either side of the mouth at the base of the tongue. The tonsils redden, swell, and are flecked with pus (left), and the throat feels sore. The surrounding glands may also become swollen and tender.

Laryngitis
Infection of the larynx. The inflammation causes hoarseness, and sometimes loss of voice.

Pharyngitis
Acute inflammation of the pharynx. The throat becomes red and raw and feels sore. Pharyngitis may also cause difficulty swallowing.

INFLUENZA

Like the cold, influenza is a viral illness, but is not nearly as common, except during epidemics. In fact, most people suffer no more than four attacks of flu during their lifetime. Influenza is generally more serious than a cold: the symptoms are worse and the complications are potentially more dangerous.

The initial symptoms of flu are similar to those of a feverish cold, but as the illness progresses it produces headaches, muscular aches and pains, a dry cough, sharp chest pains, and severe tiredness. There is no specific treatment for flu, although bed rest, plenty of fluids, and aspirin or acetaminophen will help alleviate your symptoms. If symptoms do not improve after 3 days, or if you become breathless, notify your doctor.

The main risk of an attack of flu is that the virus may spread to cause bronchitis or pneumonia. If you already have a chronic chest disease or suffer from heart or kidney disease, seek medical advice when your flu symptoms first appear.

WARNING
Flu can sometimes have serious complications. Seek medical advice when flu symptoms first appear in:
♦ The elderly or the very ill
♦ Those suffering from chronic lung, heart, or kidney disease
♦ The very young

INFLUENZA : THE INSIDE STORY

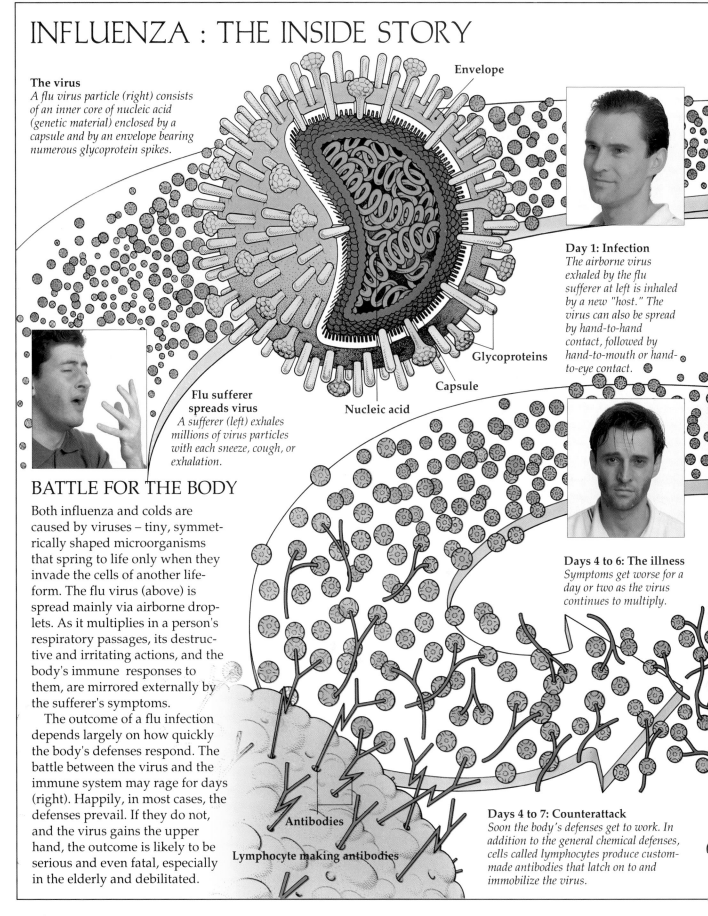

The virus
A flu virus particle (right) consists of an inner core of nucleic acid (genetic material) enclosed by a capsule and by an envelope bearing numerous glycoprotein spikes.

Envelope

Glycoproteins

Capsule

Nucleic acid

Day 1: Infection
The airborne virus exhaled by the flu sufferer at left is inhaled by a new "host." The virus can also be spread by hand-to-hand contact, followed by hand-to-mouth or hand-to-eye contact.

Flu sufferer spreads virus
A sufferer (left) exhales millions of virus particles with each sneeze, cough, or exhalation.

Days 4 to 6: The illness
Symptoms get worse for a day or two as the virus continues to multiply.

BATTLE FOR THE BODY

Both influenza and colds are caused by viruses – tiny, symmetrically shaped microorganisms that spring to life only when they invade the cells of another lifeform. The flu virus (above) is spread mainly via airborne droplets. As it multiplies in a person's respiratory passages, its destructive and irritating actions, and the body's immune responses to them, are mirrored externally by the sufferer's symptoms.

The outcome of a flu infection depends largely on how quickly the body's defenses respond. The battle between the virus and the immune system may rage for days (right). Happily, in most cases, the defenses prevail. If they do not, and the virus gains the upper hand, the outcome is likely to be serious and even fatal, especially in the elderly and debilitated.

Antibodies

Lymphocyte making antibodies

Days 4 to 7: Counterattack
Soon the body's defenses get to work. In addition to the general chemical defenses, cells called lymphocytes produce custom-made antibodies that latch on to and immobilize the virus.

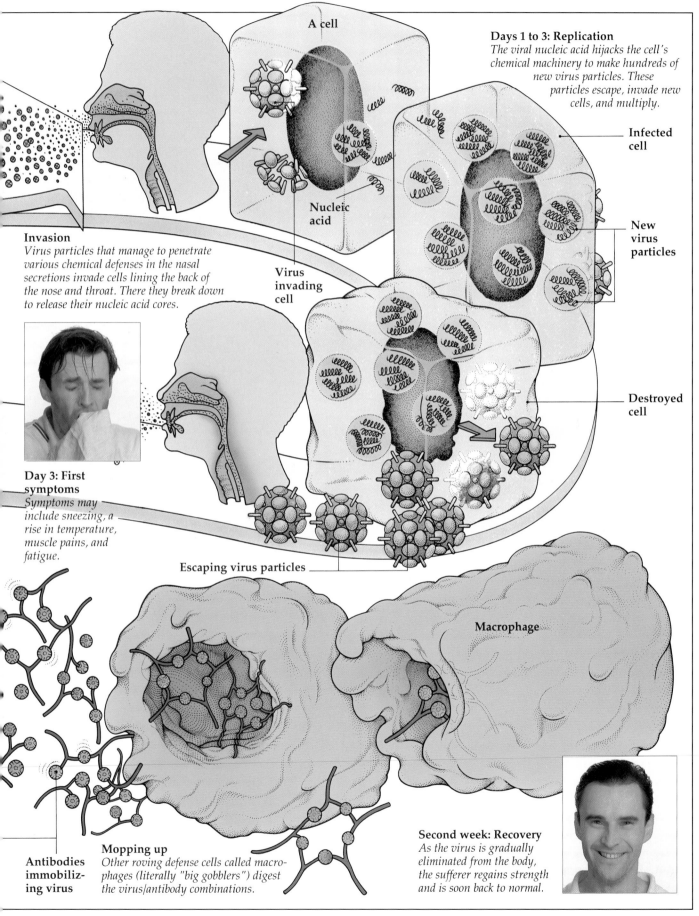

A cell

Days 1 to 3: Replication
The viral nucleic acid hijacks the cell's chemical machinery to make hundreds of new virus particles. These particles escape, invade new cells, and multiply.

Infected cell

Nucleic acid

New virus particles

Invasion
Virus particles that manage to penetrate various chemical defenses in the nasal secretions invade cells lining the back of the nose and throat. There they break down to release their nucleic acid cores.

Virus invading cell

Destroyed cell

Day 3: First symptoms
Symptoms may include sneezing, a rise in temperature, muscle pains, and fatigue.

Escaping virus particles

Macrophage

Antibodies immobilizing virus

Mopping up
Other roving defense cells called macrophages (literally "big gobblers") digest the virus/antibody combinations.

Second week: Recovery
As the virus is gradually eliminated from the body, the sufferer regains strength and is soon back to normal.

COUGHS AND SORE THROATS

Coughing caused by inflammation or irritation of the respiratory tract is one of the most common symptoms of illness. A cough may develop during any common respiratory infection, such as a cold, influenza, or bronchitis, but may also result from irritation of the air passages caused by inhaling smoke or other pollutants. Some chronic chest diseases also produce a cough, which may be the first symptom of a serious condition such as tuberculosis or lung cancer.

Another condition that often accompanies a cold or bout of flu is a sore throat. There are two types: pharyngitis, a mild inflammation of the back of the throat, and tonsillitis, a more severe inflammation of the tonsils. Both can be caused by a viral or bacterial infection.

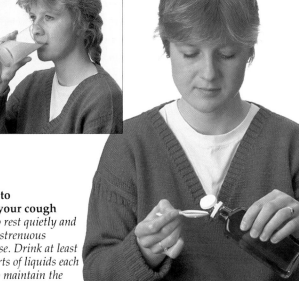

How to ease your cough
Try to rest quietly and avoid strenuous exercise. Drink at least 2 quarts of liquids each day to maintain the fluidity of your bronchial secretions. If you find that it helps, take the recommended dose of an over-the-counter cough medicine.

The best treatment for either condition is to drink plenty of fluids, to suck throat lozenges, and, if the pain is severe, to take aspirin (children under 16 should *not* take aspirin) or acetaminophen. Mouthwashes, gargles, or throat sprays may also soothe your throat. However, if your symptoms persist for more than a few days, consult your doctor.

HELPLINE
COUGHING

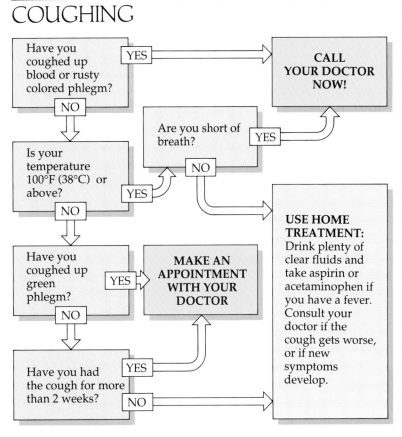

Have you coughed up blood or rusty colored phlegm? — YES → **CALL YOUR DOCTOR NOW!**

NO ↓

Is your temperature 100°F (38°C) or above? — YES →

Are you short of breath? — YES → **CALL YOUR DOCTOR NOW!**

NO

NO ↓

Have you coughed up green phlegm? — YES → **MAKE AN APPOINTMENT WITH YOUR DOCTOR**

NO ↓

Have you had the cough for more than 2 weeks? — YES → **MAKE AN APPOINTMENT WITH YOUR DOCTOR**

NO →

USE HOME TREATMENT: Drink plenty of clear fluids and take aspirin or acetaminophen if you have a fever. Consult your doctor if the cough gets worse, or if new symptoms develop.

FEVER

A rise in body temperature, a fever, is part of the body's mechanism for fighting infection. A fever often accompanies a cold or bout of flu and is not in itself serious if you have been otherwise healthy, unless your temperature rises above 104°F (40°C). However, if a child has a temperature above 102°F (39°C), or an adult has a temperature above 104°F (40°C), tell your doctor as soon as possible about the temperature and any other symptoms. You should also seek medical advice if a raised temperature persists for more than 48 hours.

With a feverish illness you should avoid wrapping up with extra blankets

CHOOSING THE RIGHT REMEDY

Every year we spend several hundred million dollars on over-the-counter preparations for the treatment of cold and flu symptoms. Most are moderately effective, although none can alter the course of the illness. When shopping for a medicine, always look at the list of active ingredients. The main ingredient is usually a pain-relieving analgesic, which is often combined with a decongestant and an antihistamine to relieve a blocked-up nose and sneezing. Cough remedies usually contain antitussives to suppress a cough or expectorants to loosen mucus in the airways. Most doctors recommend that you take preparations containing only ingredients that will relieve your particular symptoms, rather than a "cocktail" of agents designed to treat the whole range of possible symptoms.

in an overheated room. Sponge your body with lukewarm water or rubbing alcohol to help keep it cool and comfortable. Medication such as aspirin (children under the age of 16 should *not* take aspirin) or acetaminophen will help reduce the temperature.

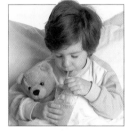

Dealing with a high temperature

The feverish patient is hot, flushed, and sweats more than usual. To reduce the temperature, and make the patient feel more comfortable, sponge his or her legs, arms, neck, and face with lukewarm water. Allow the skin to dry naturally; the evaporation of the water will cool the body.

Because sweating increases the patient's thirst, it is important to provide frequent cold drinks.

ASK YOUR DOCTOR COLDS AND FLU

Q My sister-in-law has bronchitis and has recently been immunized against flu. Should my whole family be immunized? If so, how long would immunity last?

A Most doctors recommend immunization only for people who are particularly susceptible to flu, or for those who are at special risk from complications of the illness. This includes the elderly, and people like your sister-in-law who suffer from chronic medical conditions such as bronchitis, emphysema, kidney disease, or heart disease. The vaccine has only a short action, and needs to be repeated every year.

Q Should children who suffer from recurrent sore throats have their tonsils removed?

A Usually not. If the sore throats are caused by true tonsillitis, then tonsillectomy may be considered, particularly if the infections are frequent or affect the child's general health. However, within a year or so, attacks usually become less frequent, so doctors often treat the infections with antibiotics and wait for a natural improvement in symptoms.

Q Is it possible to catch a cold or flu by shaking hands with a person who is already infected?

A Yes, there is evidence to show that the cold and flu viruses can be transmitted from one person to another via the hands, but you are far more likely to catch a cold or flu through "droplet infection." This method of transmission occurs when a person breathes in a virus that has been sneezed or exhaled into the air by an infected person.

HEADACHE

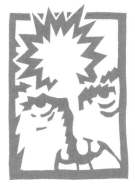

ONLY ONE PERSON in 50 has never experienced a headache. The rest of us are all too familiar with pains in the region of the forehead, at the back of the head and neck, or over the whole scalp. A persistent, disabling headache is rare, however. When a headache continues to be the only symptom over months or years, it is seldom an indication of a serious underlying disease.

The pain that we call "headache" does not originate in the brain itself, for the brain has no receptors with which to signal pain to us. A headache is most often caused by the stretching, inflammation, or spasm that can occur in the scalp, the membranes that cover the brain, and the muscles of the face and jaw, or by constriction and dilation of the blood vessels that supply the brain.

TENSION HEADACHES

Tension headaches are the most common type of headaches. "Tension" may refer to the muscular contraction around the neck, face, and head that sometimes occurs or to the psychological state of the person. Headaches can develop at any time of day and frequently last for weeks,

TENSION HEADACHES

Tension headaches are caused by tension in the muscles of the head and neck.

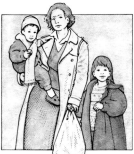

Whether you spend your time at home with demanding children or work long hours at a computer screen, the stresses of your day can cause tension in the muscles of your head and neck and thus bring on a tension headache.

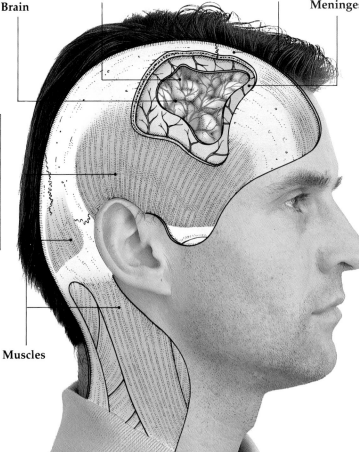

Blood vessels

Brain

Skull

Meninges

Muscles

VASCULAR HEADACHES

Vascular headaches are caused by changes in the blood vessels that supply the brain and scalp.

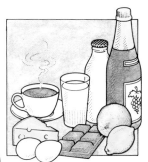

Vascular headaches may have a relationship to emotional stress. In other cases, certain foods, including dairy products, chocolate, coffee, eggs, and citrus fruits, may trigger vascular headaches.

MONITOR YOUR SYMPTOMS
HEADACHE

Most headaches develop gradually and then vanish after a few hours. Any headache that is severe, that lasts for more than 24 hours, or that recurs every few days or more frequently should always be mentioned to your doctor.

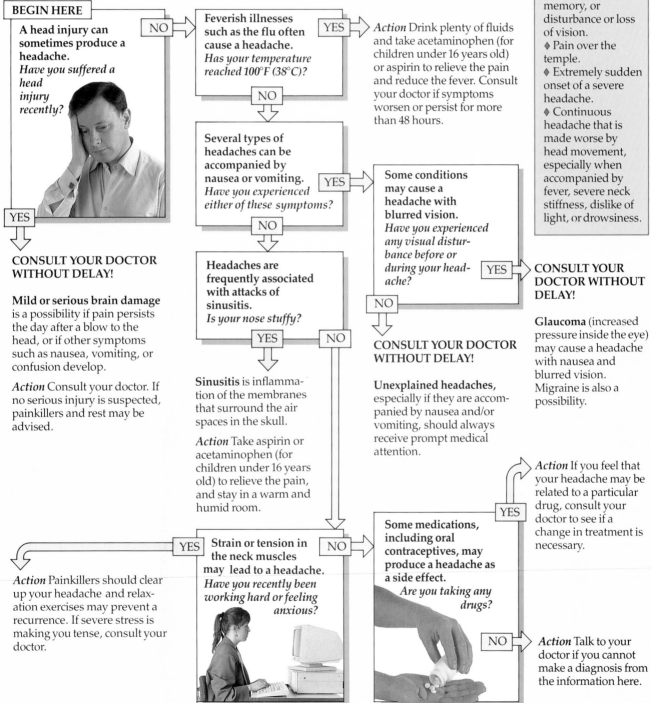

BEGIN HERE

A head injury can sometimes produce a headache.
Have you suffered a head injury recently?

NO →

Feverish illnesses such as the flu often cause a headache.
Has your temperature reached 100°F (38°C)?

YES →

Action Drink plenty of fluids and take acetaminophen (for children under 16 years old) or aspirin to relieve the pain and reduce the fever. Consult your doctor if symptoms worsen or persist for more than 48 hours.

NO ↓

Several types of headaches can be accompanied by nausea or vomiting.
Have you experienced either of these symptoms?

YES →

Some conditions may cause a headache with blurred vision.
Have you experienced any visual disturbance before or during your headache?

YES →

NO ↓

Headaches are frequently associated with attacks of sinusitis.
Is your nose stuffy?

YES ↓   NO →

YES ↓ (left side)

CONSULT YOUR DOCTOR WITHOUT DELAY!

Mild or serious brain damage is a possibility if pain persists the day after a blow to the head, or if other symptoms such as nausea, vomiting, or confusion develop.

Action Consult your doctor. If no serious injury is suspected, painkillers and rest may be advised.

Sinusitis is inflammation of the membranes that surround the air spaces in the skull.

Action Take aspirin or acetaminophen (for children under 16 years old) to relieve the pain, and stay in a warm and humid room.

CONSULT YOUR DOCTOR WITHOUT DELAY!

Unexplained headaches, especially if they are accompanied by nausea and/or vomiting, should always receive prompt medical attention.

CONSULT YOUR DOCTOR WITHOUT DELAY!

Glaucoma (increased pressure inside the eye) may cause a headache with nausea and blurred vision. Migraine is also a possibility.

YES ← | **Strain or tension in the neck muscles may lead to a headache.** *Have you recently been working hard or feeling anxious?* | NO →

Action Painkillers should clear up your headache and relaxation exercises may prevent a recurrence. If severe stress is making you tense, consult your doctor.

Some medications, including oral contraceptives, may produce a headache as a side effect.
Are you taking any drugs?

YES →

Action If you feel that your headache may be related to a particular drug, consult your doctor to see if a change in treatment is necessary.

NO →

Action Talk to your doctor if you cannot make a diagnosis from the information here.

WARNING

Consult your doctor without delay if you have:

♦ A severe headache upon waking.
♦ Any headache accompanied by vomiting, confusion, loss of memory, or disturbance or loss of vision.
♦ Pain over the temple.
♦ Extremely sudden onset of a severe headache.
♦ Continuous headache that is made worse by head movement, especially when accompanied by fever, severe neck stiffness, dislike of light, or drowsiness.

HOW TO PREVENT A HEADACHE

The following measures are worth trying if you suffer from headaches:
♦ Try to identify the cause of the headache. If it is caused by some form of stress, try not to respond to the headache by becoming more tense.
♦ If your headaches are alcohol-related, reduce your alcohol consumption or eliminate it altogether.
♦ Practice the relaxation exercises on pages 22 and 23.

months, or even years. The pain is most commonly steady, felt on both sides of the head, and located around the temples or at the back of the head and neck. It is sometimes described as a pressure, tightness, or band around the head. In rare cases, some people experience vomiting or intolerance to light (photophobia).

Although in some instances these headaches seem to be caused by muscle contraction or depression and anxiety, the origin of most is not yet understood.

VASCULAR HEADACHES

Vascular headaches are caused by temporary changes in the diameter of the blood vessels that supply the brain and scalp. Migraine is the classic vascular headache, but an alcoholic hangover headache may be another variety.

Alcohol brings on a headache by dilating the arteries in the brain and scalp. A headache can also result from the toxic effects of alcoholic drinks. Some researchers believe that the congeners used in the manufacturing process of alcohol are as important in causing headache as the ethyl alcohol itself.

What is migraine?

A migraine attack begins with a temporary narrowing, or spasm, of some of the arteries on one side of the brain. The spasm may last for up to 30 minutes and is sometimes accompanied by a disturbance in vision. Symptoms such as tingling, numbness, or weakness in one half of the body, or in both hands and around the mouth, may occur if other parts of the brain are affected.

As the spasm passes, other arteries dilate and the nerve endings in their walls are stretched, bringing on the headache pain. The pain is severe and throbbing, and there is often nausea, vomiting, sweating, fatigue, and acute sensitivity to bright light. The attack may last from a few hours to a day or two.

HOW TO RELIEVE A HEADACHE

♦ Take a warm bath to relieve tension.
♦ Take the recommended dose of aspirin or an aspirin substitute.
♦ Rest in a quiet, darkened room.
♦ Consult your doctor if these measures fail to reduce the pain or if pain is still present the following day.

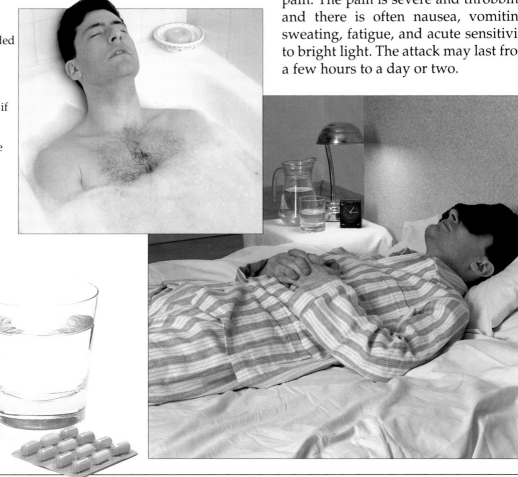

CASE HISTORY
HEADACHE AND VISUAL DISTURBANCE

WHILE STUDYING in her room one afternoon, Janine found that she was able to see less and less of the pages in the book open in front of her. Although her vision was soon back to normal, she then developed a severe headache on one side of her head. Janine began to get very concerned and wondered if she was losing her sight. After talking to her mother, she decided to call her doctor to schedule an appointment the next day.

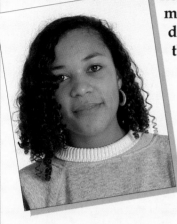

PERSONAL DETAILS
Name Janine Markson
Age 18
Occupation College student
Family No one suffers from a serious medical condition, although Janine's father has occasional headaches.

MEDICAL BACKGROUND
Janine has been free from major illness since infancy, having suffered nothing more than the usual childhood illnesses. She is a quiet, intelligent, hard-working, young woman.

THE CONSULTATION
Janine is very worried. She tells her doctor that she had lost part of her vision the previous afternoon. By closing one eye at a time, she had found that a defect – a small, sparkling area to the right of her point of focus – was present in each eye.

Going over the events of that day, Janine realizes that she had felt strange since getting up. She also mentions to her doctor that her menstrual period is due any day. After lunch, before settling down to read, she had recited some Shakespeare aloud. She had noticed that, although she could remember the sense of the passages, she sometimes had difficulty finding the right words. Then, following her disturb-ing loss of vision while reading, she had developed a bad headache on one side of her head. Otherwise, she had felt reasonably well, and her vision had returned to normal after about half an hour.

THE DIAGNOSIS
Janine's symptoms point unequivocally to an attack of CLASSIC MIGRAINE. In the morning, when she felt elated and energetic, Janine was experiencing the aura that sometimes precedes a migraine. Later on, narrowing occurred in some of the arteries supplying the left side of the back part of her brain. This affected the fibers that connect the left part of the brain with the retinas of both eyes, producing a defect in the right field of vision of both eyes.

THE TREATMENT
Brief disturbance of brain function due to a temporary reduction of blood supply is common. While it may be frightening to experience, it need not cause anxiety. Migraine attacks of this kind are usually both infrequent and unpredictable, and thus require treatment only when they occur. Doctors recommend preventive treatment only when attacks occur once a week or more. Janine's doctor prescribes a drug known to be effective for migraine.

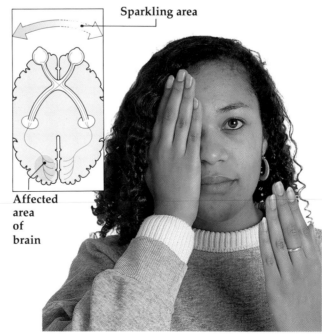

Sparkling area

Affected area of brain

Visual disturbance
The sparkling area was the result of some arterial narrowing that affected the visual fibers in the left side of the back part of her brain (red fibers in inset diagram). These fibers carry information, from the retinas of both eyes, about the right field of vision.

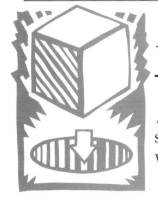

ABNORMAL BEHAVIOR

B EHAVIOR IS AS variable as each of our personalities. Some people are naturally more subdued or more forgetful, while others are more lively or excitable. However, a radical change in a person's pattern of behavior can be alarming. What could it mean and when should you do something about it?

If a member of your family is behaving in an odd manner, there are several points to consider when assessing the situation and deciding what action to take.

First, is the affected person in a suitable frame of mind to discuss the problem? There may be a clear-cut explanation for his or her change in behavior, and it is useful to ask the person some questions before you call for help.

Also consider whether the behavior is getting worse or is likely to cause harm to the person or to others. If the answer is "yes," some form of prompt action is obviously necessary.

The chart on the opposite page lists common examples of changed or worrisome behavior; it also suggests some possible courses of action. Some behavior requires emergency medical attention, while other behavior calls for a more watchful approach. Some of the major causes of disturbed behavior are discussed in this section.

Teenage moodiness
Sullen, withdrawn, or other odd behavior in a teenager is very common and often is due to anxieties about relationships or schoolwork. It should not be a cause for concern unless it persists or there are grounds for suspecting drug or alcohol abuse.

ALCOHOL AND DRUG ABUSE

Alcohol intoxication is a common cause of abusive and aggressive behavior. Persistent use of alcohol can lead to moodiness, depression, memory loss, poor school or job performance, and health problems, such as gastritis, liver disease, and high blood pressure. Remember, however, that overt signs of intoxication, including an unsteady gait and slurred speech, may be absent in the chronic heavy drinker because of the development of tolerance to alcohol.

If the drinking episodes recur frequently, try reasoning with the person when he or she is sober. Alcoholism treatment specialists, who are experienced in the process of confrontation and intervention, often are the best people to persuade the drinker that he or she needs help.

Could drugs be the cause?

The effects of drug abuse vary according to the drug being used, but possible signs include periods of dreaminess, drowsiness, confusion, hyperactivity, or partly suppressed excitement. Snorting solvents, cocaine, or heroin causes soreness around the nose or constant sniffling. Injecting drugs leaves marks on the arms.

Be sure you have proof before accusing any young person of abusing drugs. Many teenagers who have never used drugs go through a phase of being moody, dreamy, or disagreeable.

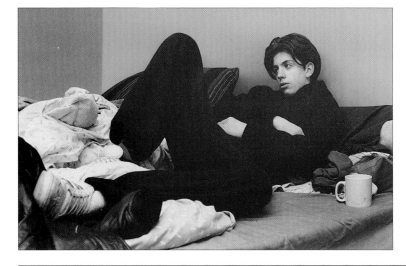

WHAT ACTION SHOULD I TAKE?

	BEHAVIOR	POSSIBLE CAUSES	ACTION
	Sudden, deepening drowsiness	Drug overdose Head injury Stroke or other brain disorder	Call a doctor or ambulance immediately.
	Recurrent drowsiness	Insufficient sleep Physical disease Heavy use of alcohol Overuse of tranquilizers Abuse of illicit drugs Depression	If lack of sleep seems unlikely and you suspect the use of alcohol or other drugs, discuss the situation with family first, then with the individual (when he or she is sober and alert), and with your doctor if necessary.
	Confusion and muddled thinking	Alcohol or drug abuse Feverish illness Severe anxiety or depression Alzheimer's disease, hardening of arteries in brain, or a heart, lung, or kidney disorder (especially in an elderly person)	If alcohol or drug abuse is suspected, take the action above. If the patient has a fever, call a doctor immediately. If you suspect a depressive illness, persuade the person to seek medical help. An elderly, confused person should undergo a complete physical examination.
	Repetitive behavior (e.g., constant hand-washing)	Possible onset of obsessional neurosis	Persuade the person to see a doctor if the behavior is seriously interfering with his or her day-to-day functioning.
	Unprovoked aggression and shouting	Alcohol or drug abuse Onset of major mental illness or physical brain disorder	Do not argue or disagree with the person. Summon a doctor and, if necessary, the police.
	Not eating	Fussy eating habits Anorexia nervosa in a teenager or young adult Severe anxiety or depression	Be concerned only if the person is losing weight or seems depressed, in which case, consult your doctor.
	Moodiness and irritability	Problems of adolescence Onset of menopause or male "midlife crisis" Common frustrations and stresses of living Depression Severe anxiety	Discuss the problems with the individual. Generally, there is no cause for medical concern unless the moodiness is persistent and has no obvious cause. Menopausal women may benefit from hormone replacement therapy and psychotherapy.
	Extreme withdrawal	Possible onset of schizophrenia or other mental disorder in a teenager or young adult Alcohol abuse Depression	Discuss the situation with your doctor.

PHYSICAL AND MENTAL ILLNESS

Physical illness can cause strange behavior. For example, sudden confusion in a child may be triggered by a fever. Likewise, you should never assume that confusion in an older person is caused by dementia until other physical illnesses have been ruled out by your doctor.

In some cases a change in behavior signals the onset of a true mental illness. Sometimes the person remains rational much of the time and can be persuaded to seek help. However, a profoundly disturbed person may refuse to consider treatment. Ask your family doctor for the name of a psychiatrist and call the police immediately if you feel threatened in any way.

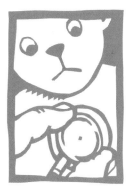

COMMON CHILDHOOD ILLNESSES

EVERY PARENT knows that children get sick. It helps to know that the majority of common illnesses that children bring home are minor and don't last long. Many illnesses that were once common, such as measles, mumps, rubella (German measles), and whooping cough, are now rare because of immunization.

Most children have at least one feverish illness in which they develop a rash of some kind. All children have sore throats, get colds, and have earaches, and most have occasional diarrhea.

COLDS, COUGHS, AND WHEEZING

Minor colds and sore throats generally require no specific treatment other than taking steps to reduce fever (see MANAGING A FEVER on page 58). Ear infections are a common complication of colds in young children (see EARACHE on page 100).

Tonsillitis
The child with tonsillitis usually has a fever, complains of a sore throat, and is generally miserable. The tonsils are red, swollen, and may have specks of yellow pus on them.

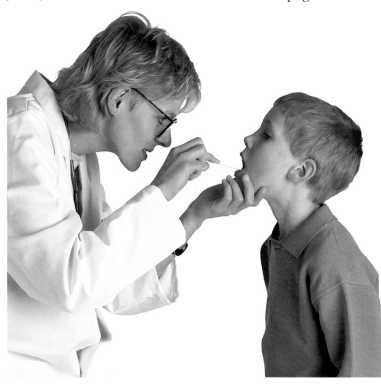

Coughs

A child with cold symptoms may develop a barking cough, hoarseness, and a strange, crowing, breathing sound. This is croup, which often is due to a viral infection. Croup causes narrowing of the upper part of the airway. An effective home remedy for croup is steam or moist air inhalation, which can be achieved by using vaporizers or by standing the child in a closed bathroom with the shower running. Sometimes going outside to breathe cool night air will suffice. Croup usually goes away on its own after several days, but some children develop serious breathing difficulties, in which case you should call your doctor.

Whooping cough starts with a runny nose and a slight temperature followed by bouts of severe coughing, during which you will hear the characteristic "whoop." It is one of the more dangerous childhood diseases, and vaccination provides valuable protection.

Wheezing

About one in 10 children has recurrent bouts of wheezing, which may be caused by asthma. Most children grow out of asthma; in the meantime, it can usually be treated by medication and by avoiding the substances that trigger it.

Bronchiolitis is caused by a viral infection of the airways. The main symptoms are cough, rapid breathing, difficulty eating, and wheezing. Bronchiolitis can be a serious condition.

RASHES

Illnesses that produce an infectious or noninfectious rash on the body are commonplace in childhood.

Infectious rashes

One common cause of rash is chickenpox. Up to 21 days (the usual time is 7 to 14 days) after contact with a person who is infected with the virus, the child develops a rash, mainly on the trunk. The rash starts as crops of pimples, which then become blisterlike and eventually form crusts. The inside of the mouth, eyes, or nose may also be affected and the child often has a fever. The rash, which lasts about a week and then gradually fades, can be very itchy and may be soothed by calamine lotion, oatmeal baths, or prescription medicines.

Roseola is another common illness that most often affects children under 2 and is probably caused by a virus. The child develops a high temperature that lasts for 3 or 4 days. As the temperature drops, a rash appears on the body, where it is visible for a few hours or days.

Fifth disease (also called slapped cheek disease) is also a common infectious rash that is caused by a virus. The main feature is a red rash on the cheeks, which lasts for about a week to 10 days.

Noninfectious rashes

Some rashes are not caused by infections; a common example is eczema. The eczema rash is scaly, red, and itchy, often occurring on the face, in the elbow creases, and behind the knees. It is not unusual for a child with eczema also to suffer from asthma or hay fever. There may also be a history of these conditions, all of which are probably caused by allergies, in other members of the family. Children with eczema tend to have very dry skin, which should be moisturized regularly. The child's doctor may also recommend a short course of treatment with corticosteroid creams.

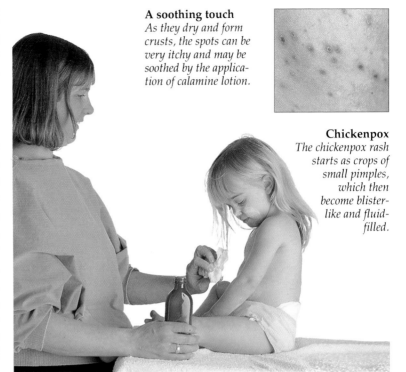

A soothing touch
As they dry and form crusts, the spots can be very itchy and may be soothed by the application of calamine lotion.

Chickenpox
The chickenpox rash starts as crops of small pimples, which then become blisterlike and fluidfilled.

HOW TO PREVENT DIAPER RASH

Diaper rash is often caused by the irritant effect of urine and stool on the skin. Basic preventive treatment includes frequent diaper changes, thorough washing and drying at each diaper change, the use of a protective barrier cream, and allowing your baby to go diaperless as much as possible during the day.

A diaper rash that does not clear up within a few days may be caused by simple skin inflammation or dermatitis, or by the fungal infection thrush. These forms of diaper rash may require treatment by your baby's pediatrician.

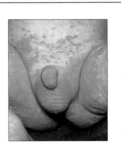

Diaper rash
Severe diaper rash can be very sore and uncomfortable for a baby.

Prevention
You can prevent diaper rash from occurring by keeping your baby's skin dry, clean, and exposed to the air for as long as possible each day. Frequent changes and careful cleaning will help you prevent the problem.

MONITOR YOUR SYMPTOMS
SLEEPING PROBLEMS IN CHILDREN

Children 1 year old or older usually sleep through the night without disruption. The amount of sleep a child needs varies from about 9 hours or less to 12 hours. Sleeping difficulties, such as refusal to go to sleep or frequent waking during the night, can have several possible causes.

WARNING

It is very important not to let sleep problems get out of hand. They must be dealt with promptly as soon as they appear, before they are allowed to become established. Any sleeping problem is more difficult to deal with once it has become a habit.

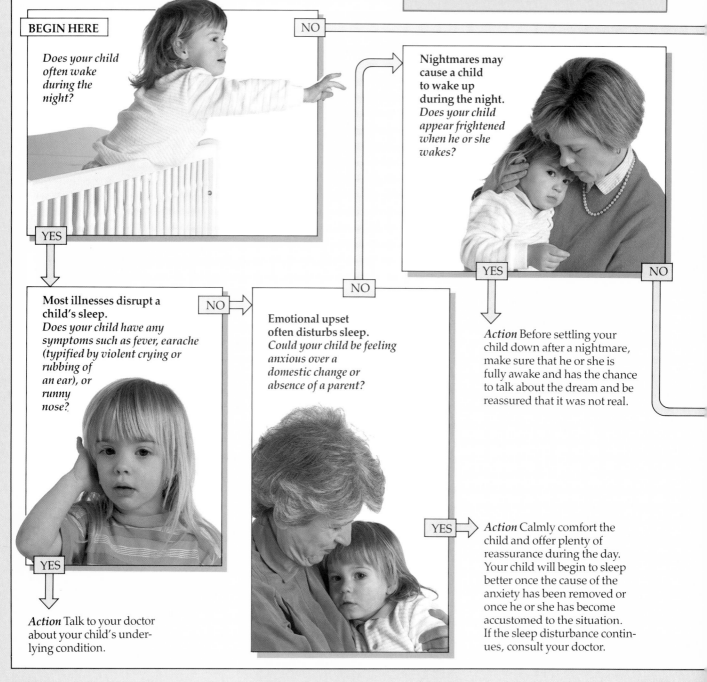

BEGIN HERE

Does your child often wake during the night?

NO

Nightmares may cause a child to wake up during the night. *Does your child appear frightened when he or she wakes?*

YES · NO

YES

Most illnesses disrupt a child's sleep. *Does your child have any symptoms such as fever, earache (typified by violent crying or rubbing of an ear), or runny nose?*

NO

Emotional upset often disturbs sleep. *Could your child be feeling anxious over a domestic change or absence of a parent?*

Action Before settling your child down after a nightmare, make sure that he or she is fully awake and has the chance to talk about the dream and be reassured that it was not real.

YES

Action Talk to your doctor about your child's underlying condition.

YES

Action Calmly comfort the child and offer plenty of reassurance during the day. Your child will begin to sleep better once the cause of the anxiety has been removed or once he or she has become accustomed to the situation. If the sleep disturbance continues, consult your doctor.

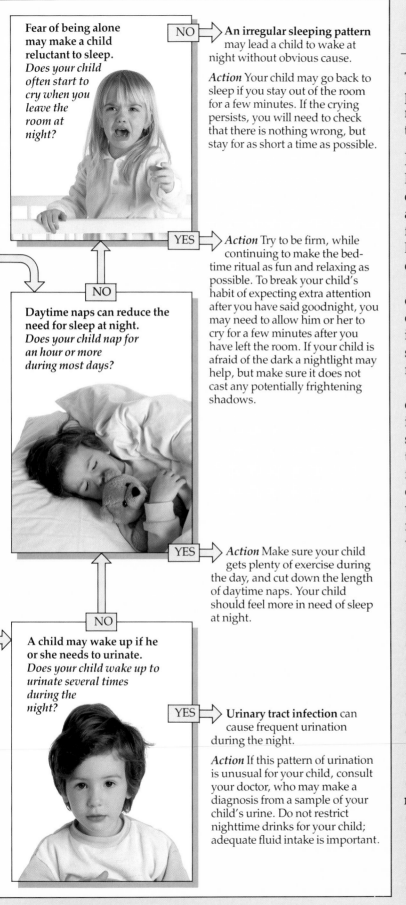

Fear of being alone may make a child reluctant to sleep. *Does your child often start to cry when you leave the room at night?*

NO → **An irregular sleeping pattern** may lead a child to wake at night without obvious cause.

Action Your child may go back to sleep if you stay out of the room for a few minutes. If the crying persists, you will need to check that there is nothing wrong, but stay for as short a time as possible.

YES → *Action* Try to be firm, while continuing to make the bedtime ritual as fun and relaxing as possible. To break your child's habit of expecting extra attention after you have said goodnight, you may need to allow him or her to cry for a few minutes after you have left the room. If your child is afraid of the dark a nightlight may help, but make sure it does not cast any potentially frightening shadows.

Daytime naps can reduce the need for sleep at night. *Does your child nap for an hour or more during most days?*

YES → *Action* Make sure your child gets plenty of exercise during the day, and cut down the length of daytime naps. Your child should feel more in need of sleep at night.

A child may wake up if he or she needs to urinate. *Does your child wake up to urinate several times during the night?*

YES → **Urinary tract infection** can cause frequent urination during the night.

Action If this pattern of urination is unusual for your child, consult your doctor, who may make a diagnosis from a sample of your child's urine. Do not restrict nighttime drinks for your child; adequate fluid intake is important.

FEEDING, DIGESTIVE, AND BLADDER PROBLEMS

There are several other common health problems in childhood that are usually minor and of short duration. However, they can cause anxiety for parents.

Feeding problems

Feeding problems are common, especially in early infancy, while weaning, and during the toddler stage. Food refusal, for example, requires patience. Make sure the older child is not filling up on junk food or soda pop between meals.

If the problem persists, consult your doctor or pediatrician, especially if your child is not growing properly or is vomiting repeatedly. Vomiting may be a symptom of disease or may occur as a result of crying or emotional distress.

Infections of the gastrointestinal tract often cause diarrhea and vomiting. It is important to give a child with these symptoms plenty of fluids. Gastroenteritis can be serious, particularly in infants and babies, who can easily become dehydrated. If symptoms do not clear up quickly, consult your doctor, who may recommend that you treat your child with oral rehydration solutions.

Bed-wetting

Bed-wetting is common in otherwise healthy children, affecting more than 10 percent of 5 year olds and about 4 percent of 10 year olds. In most cases, bed-wetting is due to slow maturation of nervous system functions concerned with bladder control. If you are concerned that your child still wets the bed, discuss the problem with your doctor.

There are a number of ways to cope with the problem, such as lifting the child onto a potty or toilet during the night to pass urine, and rewarding him or her for dry nights. Try keeping fluid intake low from dinner until bedtime. Another useful solution is to purchase a special alarm bell that is wired to a pad on the bed. As soon as the child starts to wet the bed, the alarm sounds and the child, once awakened, can get up and go to the bathroom. This teaches the child to recognize the need to pass urine and wake up on his or her own.

Bed-wetting may indicate a urinary tract infection, particularly if your child is usually dry. Urinary tract infection is a common problem in young children, especially in girls. The urine may smell unpleasant or the child may complain of stomachache, have a fever, or just seem sick. Urinary tract infection requires medical attention because repeated infections can damage the kidneys. In the meantime, do not restrict fluid intake.

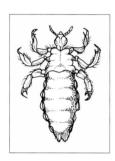

Head lice
Head lice are one of the most common childhood parasites. They infest the hair on the human head and cause the skin to itch where they bite.

Shampoo
A shampoo containing pyrethrins is the best way to treat lice. Rub it into the child's wet hair, leave for 5 to 10 minutes or according to the manufacturer's instructions, and rinse it off with clean water.

DEALING WITH PARASITES

Childhood parasites, which include lice, scabies, and pinworms, are not uncommon. Each of these infections requires treatment of the entire family.

Scabies causes an itchy, red rash. It is most common on the hands, wrists, and fingers. A prescribed lotion must be applied to the whole body below the head and neck to clear up the infestation. Pinworms cause itching around the anus, especially during the night, and may make the child very irritable. Creams or ointments can soothe anal itching. In addition, your doctor may prescribe a drug to eradicate the worms.

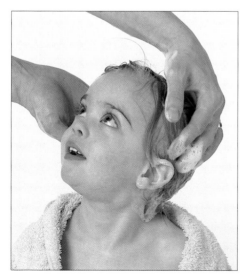

THE SICK CHILD

Babies and toddlers often show nonspecific symptoms of illness, such as lack of interest in food, excessive sleepiness, floppiness, fretfulness, and irritability. If you are worried that your child is sick, consult your doctor promptly, particularly if your child has a persistently high temperature, recurrent diarrhea or vomiting, is unusually drowsy, has a seizure, or develops an unusual swelling.

Managing a fever

If your child develops a fever, take off most of his or her clothes. Do not wrap the child in blankets – this only raises the temperature. Give plenty of clear fluids, which will prevent dehydration and may

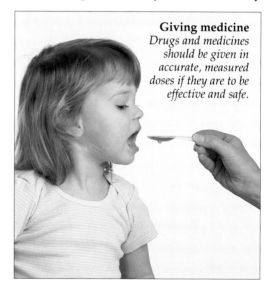

Giving medicine
Drugs and medicines should be given in accurate, measured doses if they are to be effective and safe.

help reduce the temperature. Don't worry if your child refuses to eat.

If the fever persists, give a small dose (appropriate for the child's age) of acetaminophen syrup, drops, or pills. You can repeat the dose every 4 hours for up to 24 hours. If the temperature remains high, sponge the child with lukewarm water, repeating every 2 to 4 hours if necessary. Do not use cold water; it can cause the temperature to increase. An electric fan directed toward the child will help the cooling process.

HOW TO TAKE A CHILD'S TEMPERATURE

Mercury thermometer
Place the thermometer under the tongue, ask your child to close his or her mouth, and leave the thermometer in place for 3 minutes. This type is recommended only for children who are old enough to understand that they should not bite the mercury bulb.

Strip thermometer
Hold the strip flat against your child's forehead with both hands, keeping your fingers clear of the numbered panels. Wait about 15 seconds before reading the temperature. The reading is only approximate with the strip thermometer method.

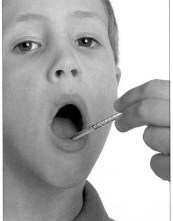

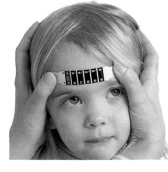

Armpit method
Sit with your child on your lap, facing away from you. Raise the child's arm, place the thermometer underneath, then bring the arm down gently on the thermometer. Leave the thermometer in place for 3 minutes. The reading will be about 1°F (0.6°C) lower than the child's actual body temperature.

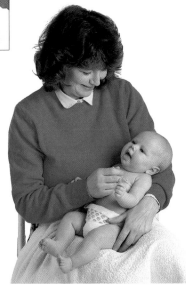

Seizures

About 3 to 5 percent of children have a seizure that is triggered by a high temperature. Children 2 to 4 years old are most often affected. If your child has a seizure, lay the child on his or her side, facing the floor. Do not put anything in the child's mouth. If your child has never had a seizure before, or if the seizure goes on for more than 5 minutes, call your doctor. Temperature control is particularly important in children who are prone to seizures initiated by a fever.

ASK YOUR DOCTOR
CHILDHOOD
PROBLEMS

Q My 5-month-old baby cries constantly every evening. Is there something wrong with her ?

A Many babies between 3 and 6 months have bouts of inconsolable crying for no apparent reason, usually in the evening. The most likely reason for this is colic, which is probably caused by painful spasmodic contractions of the bowel. There is no treatment for colic. You can try to soothe your baby by cuddling, rocking, or placing her (well supervised) on top of a running laundry dryer. Be reassured that the crying is only a phase and your baby will grow out of it.

Q Why does my child seem to get many more nosebleeds than other children his age?

A Nosebleeds are very common in childhood and often result from upper respiratory tract infections or from injury caused by a blow to the nose or by nose picking. Very dry homes can aggravate the nosebleeding that is caused by picking the nose. In most cases, the bleeding will stop quickly if you sit the child up, squeeze the nose firmly, and ask the child to breathe through his or her mouth. If your child has frequent, heavy nosebleeds, consult your doctor.

Q My 3-year-old son has only one testicle. Will the other one come down when he gets older?

A If one or both testes have not descended to the scrotum by the time a boy is a few months old, they are unlikely to do so without a simple operation (which should be done before age 5). Consult your doctor.

CHEST PAIN

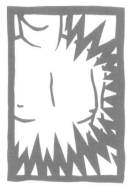

A SUDDEN PAIN in the chest, especially if it is severe, usually causes considerable alarm. "Is it a heart attack?" is often the first, panicky reaction to this symptom. The answer is most often "no." Although heart attacks are by no means rare – 1.5 million Americans have one over the course of a year – sudden chest pain is just as likely to have another, much less serious, cause.

The chest area, lying between the neck and the bottom of the rib cage, is subject to a variety of pains that stem from many different sites. Most chest pain is due to a temporary, minor problem affecting the spine or the skin, muscles, and ribs of the chest wall. Occasionally, the pain occurs because of a serious disorder of the heart or lungs. Unless the cause of any chest pain you have is immediately apparent, the best course of action is to contact your doctor for advice.

MINOR CAUSES OF CHEST PAIN

If you have strained a muscle, possibly as a result of overexercising or a severe cough, you may feel sudden, sharp pains that are made worse by movement. A disorder of the back can occasionally cause a sharp pain in the chest in addition to back pain, because some of the nerves that emerge from the spine travel around the body to the front of the chest. Inflammation of the muscles between your ribs can cause a sharp pain on one side of the chest. This condition is usually the result of a viral infection and is accompanied by other symptoms, such as a sore throat, fever, or cough. In rare cases, another viral infection, shingles, can inflame a nerve in the chest, causing a burning pain in the skin and a rash of blisters around the affected nerve.

If your chest pain is severe and persistent, it may be due to a rib that has fractured. Another possible cause is Tietze's syndrome, in which the cartilage that joins the ribs to the breastbone becomes inflamed. With both a fractured rib and Tietze's syndrome, you will feel an area of tenderness over the site of the fracture or inflammation.

If you have a strained muscle, try to avoid any movement that causes more pain. You can take aspirin or acetaminophen to help relieve the pain. A fractured rib usually heals on its own. Chest binders can be used to splint the ribs and relieve pain but they have the disadvantage of preventing complete breathing.

If you have Tietze's syndrome, your doctor will prescribe anti-inflammatory drugs to reduce the swelling.

SERIOUS CAUSES OF CHEST PAIN

Serious causes of chest pain are disorders of the heart and of the lungs. Chest pain from the heart may indicate the onset of a life-threatening condition. For this reason, it is essential that you are able to recognize the early signs of a heart attack and that you are able to distinguish them from less serious types of chest pain (see AM I HAVING A HEART ATTACK? on page 62).

Sports injuries
Injuries sustained during sports or during a fall are a common cause of chest pain. The pain may develop some time after the moment of injury. In most cases it is caused by muscular strain or damage to the rib cage. However, the possibility of damage to the lungs or heart should not be ruled out.

WHERE DOES CHEST PAIN COME FROM?

The chest contains the vital organs of the heart and lungs, lying within a strong, protective "cage" of skin, muscle, cartilage, and bone. Pain in the chest may originate in any part of the outer cage, in the membranes that line the heart and lungs, or in the vital organs themselves. Chest pain can be an important warning signal of a developing heart disease or respiratory disorder such as bronchitis or pneumonia.

SIDE VIEW OF ORGANS

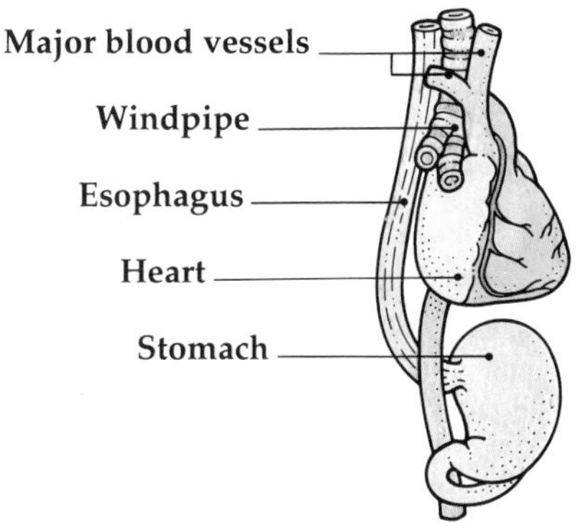

Major blood vessels

Windpipe

Esophagus

Heart

Stomach

Esophagus
This tube runs down from the throat and behind the heart to the stomach (see diagram at left). Sometimes, the lower end of the esophagus cannot prevent a backflow of acid from the stomach. The backflow of acid causes a burning sensation known as heartburn. The pain actually comes from acid in the esophagus, which lies behind the heart.

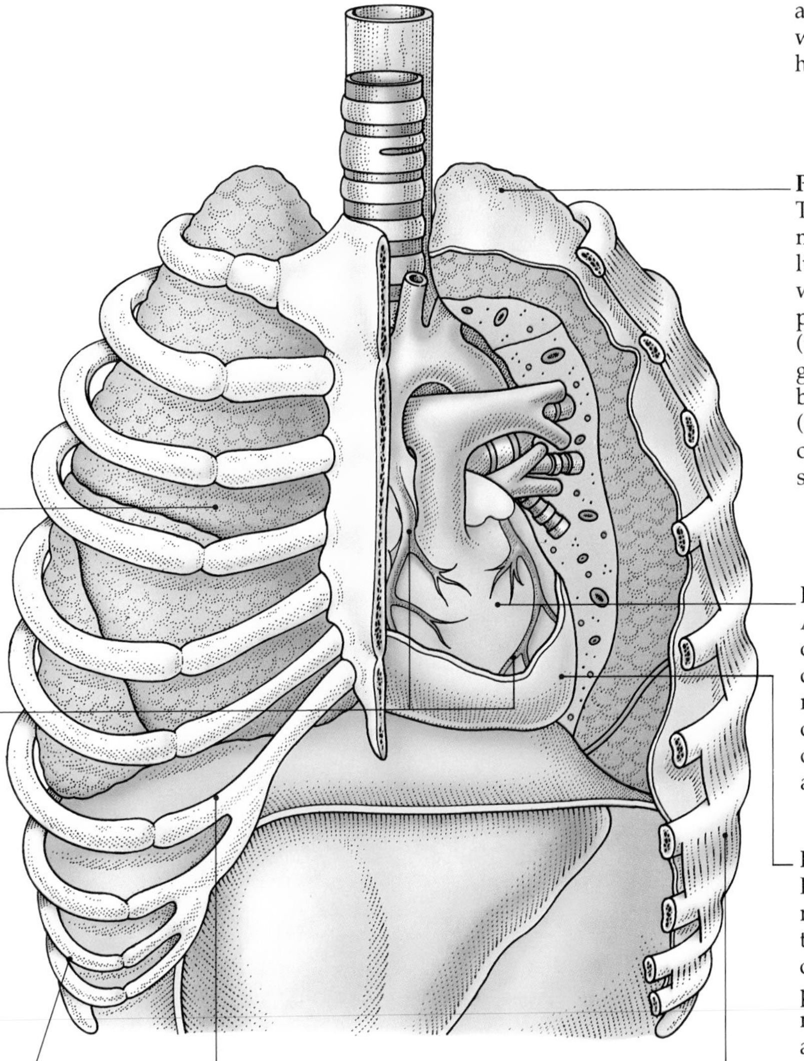

Pectoral muscles
The two main muscles of the chest wall, pectoralis major and pectoralis minor, may become strained through overuse, resulting in a short, stabbing pain.

Lung
Severe lung infection, such as bronchitis or pneumonia, can lead to chest pain and difficulty breathing.

Coronary arteries
These major vessels, which supply blood to the heart, can become narrowed by coronary heart disease. Angina (chest pain during exertion) may result because not enough oxygen, carried in the blood, can get through the arteries to the heart muscle.

Rib
A rib may be fractured by a blow or a fall, causing severe chest pain that is made worse by deep breathing.

Costal cartilage
This cartilage attaches the ribs to the breastbone; Tietze's syndrome causes tenderness and chest pain made worse by moving the arms or trunk.

Skin
A strip of skin on the chest wall may become painful and blistered as a result of shingles, a viral infection of the underlying nerves.

Pleura
The two-layered membrane lining the lungs and the chest wall can become painfully inflamed (pleurisy) or air can get into the space between the layers (pneumothorax), causing pain and shortness of breath.

Heart
A blockage in a coronary artery can deprive the heart muscle of oxygen, causing severe, crushing chest pain – a heart attack.

Pericardium
Inflammation of this membrane covering the heart, due to a chest infection, causes pain that sometimes mimics a heart attack.

Intercostal muscles
These muscles, which lie between the ribs, may become inflamed, causing sudden pain in the lower chest.

WHAT IS HEARTBURN?

Heartburn is pain in the middle of the chest that is caused by acid reflux. Reflux is a backflow of acid from the stomach into the esophagus that may be caused by overeating, by eating rich or spicy foods, by drinking alcohol, or by eating too quickly. It is more likely to occur if you lie down after a meal.

How to prevent and relieve heartburn

◊ Avoid fried and highly spiced food

◊ Eat several small meals rather than a couple of large ones

◊ Avoid alcohol

◊ Raise the head of your bed about 4 inches and sleep propped up

◊ Lose weight

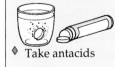

◊ Take antacids

AM I HAVING A HEART ATTACK?

A heart attack occurs when one of the coronary arteries that supplies blood to the heart becomes blocked. The pain is an immediate signal that the heart muscle is being damaged.

Anyone who suffers severe chest pain without an obvious cause should call for medical help immediately. Even if the pain seems to ease, call your doctor or go to a hospital emergency room.

You may experience:

◊ A dull, crushing pain that feels like a heavy weight in the center of the chest. The pain may spread into the neck and jaw and along the arms (see right).
◊ Nausea that may or may not be accompanied by vomiting.
◊ Severe fright and a strong sense that death is imminent.

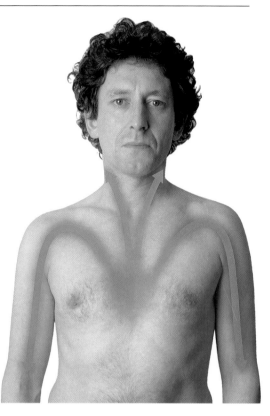

If you have chest pain that seems to come from the breastbone, jaw, neck, shoulder, arm, or upper abdomen, seek help immediately. If you are having a heart attack, lifesaving treatment must be given as early as possible.

Are all heart pains dangerous?

Not every pain in the heart area is life threatening. Sometimes, pain similar to that of a heart attack comes on during exertion and is immediately relieved by rest. In this case, the pain is known as angina pectoris (or angina). The pain results from the heart muscle receiving insufficient blood, rather than the complete lack of a blood supply that characterizes a heart attack.

Another painful disorder that can be mistaken for a heart attack is pericarditis. This is an inflammation of the pericardium, the lubricated membrane that covers the heart and allows it to beat almost without friction. However, the pain of pericarditis differs from that of a heart attack and it is usually relieved simply by leaning forward.

How do I recognize lung pain?

If you experience sudden breathlessness accompanied by a severe attack of chest pain that is worse when inhaling, the cause may be a collapsed lung. A collapsed lung may follow a chest injury, or it may be due to a weakness in the lung tissue. Another possible cause may be a blood clot in one of the lung arteries.

A sharp pain that sometimes travels to the tip of one shoulder may be caused by pleurisy, an inflammation of the membrane that covers the lungs. This pain is worse when you take a deep breath, and there are usually other symptoms, such as a loose cough and yellow sputum. Pleurisy usually results from a severe chest infection, such as bronchitis or pneumonia. It can be life threatening, particularly in the elderly.

A rare cause of persistent chest pain is a lung tumor that is pressing on a rib or stretching the lining of the lung. However, pain from a lung tumor tends to be accompanied by another symptom, such as a cough, weight loss, or coughing up blood.

INVESTIGATING CHEST PAIN

When you see your doctor about any suspicious chest pain, he or she will need to know whether you have other symptoms such as a cough or difficulty breathing. Your doctor will listen to your heart and lungs with a stethoscope, and then measure your pulse and blood pressure. You may also have a chest X-ray and an electrocardiogram (ECG).

How is chest pain treated?

The treatment of serious causes of chest pain depends on the diagnosis. If coronary heart disease is responsible for your angina or heart attack, you may be prescribed drugs to improve the flow of blood to the heart muscle. In severe cases, you may need balloon angioplasty or a coronary artery bypass operation to treat a narrowed or blocked coronary artery.

A collapsed lung often heals on its own within a few days, but if it is severe you may need to have a tube inserted to reinflate it. If you have pleurisy due to a lung infection, your doctor may prescribe antibiotics and anti-inflammatory drugs. Lung cancer is treated by surgery, radiation therapy, or chemotherapy.

The electrocardiogram
Your doctor may perform this test to check the health of your heart. As you exercise, your heart rate and the electrical activity of your heart are measured via electrodes.

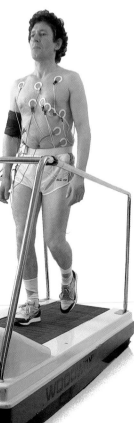

EMERGENCY TREATMENT

If someone in your family suddenly develops severe chest pain, call for medical help immediately. While waiting for help to arrive, loosen any tight clothing around the chest and neck, and stay as calm as possible. If breathing stops, lay the person on a hard, flat surface and start mouth-to-mouth resuscitation; if you cannot feel a pulse, begin cardiopulmonary resuscitation (CPR, see page 130).

ASK YOUR DOCTOR
CHEST PAIN

Q Recently, my heart has suddenly started beating very quickly. I feel breathless and have pains in my chest. My doctor says that I am healthy, so what could be wrong with me?

A Your attacks are probably due to anxiety or tension. People who feel anxious tend to hyperventilate – that is, their breathing becomes abnormally shallow and rapid. This leads to loss of carbon dioxide from the blood, which in turn causes the symptoms you describe. Minimize any obvious causes of stress in your life, and try some deep breathing exercises.

Q I occasionally suffer from a sudden attack of sharp chest pain that lasts a few seconds and feels like a knife has been stuck into me. Is this a warning of an impending heart attack?

A Sharp, stabbing, brief chest pain has none of the features of pain originating from the heart. The cause of the pain that you describe is not known. If you would like further reassurance, talk to your doctor about this chest pain.

Q Last year my severe chest pain was diagnosed as a "small heart attack." What does this mean?

A During a heart attack, the heart muscle is damaged by deprivation of oxygen. A "small heart attack" is a vague term that may imply that only a small area of the muscle has been damaged and the normal function of your heart has not been significantly impaired.

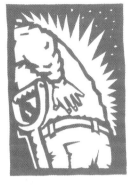

BACK PAIN

Almost all of us suffer from back pain at some time in our lives – it is the largest single cause of time off from work in the US. Fortunately, most people are in discomfort for only a few days and, with appropriate rest and pain relief, are soon back to their normal daily routine at home and at work.

Why is back pain so common? To understand the problem, it is necessary to know something about the spine, a complex structure of interlocking bones, cartilage, and muscles (see below and right).

THE STRUCTURE OF THE SPINE

The spine consists of a column of 24 bones, called vertebrae, that are separated by shock-absorbing and load-bearing discs formed of tough cartilage. At the rear of each vertebra are seven protruding knobs, called vertebral processes. Four of the processes fit together to form joints with the vertebrae above and below; the other three serve as attachments

for a variety of muscles. Running through the spine is a cable of nerve tissue, the spinal cord, from which nerves emerge at regular intervals through the gaps that exist between the vertebrae.

Binding the entire spinal structure together are many powerful muscles and strong ligaments, which limit the movements we can make. The spine is most flexible and mobile in the neck region; in the chest and lower back it has less flexibility but greater stability.

Spinal cord
This cable of nerve tissue, which acts as a switching cable for nerve messages passing between different parts of the body, runs through the center of the vertebrae.

Lumbar region of the spine
Consists of five vertebrae. This is the most common region for back pain, partly because of the greater stress it bears.

Coccyx
Consists of four fused vertebrae.

Sacrum
Consists of five fused vertebrae.

Cross section of lumbar vertebra

THE SPINAL COLUMN

The spine is composed of three main sections – the cervical region at the neck, the thoracic region at the chest, and the lumbar region at the abdomen. Most backaches result from minor damage to, or misalignment of, the structures shown, or from strain on the overlying ligaments and muscles.

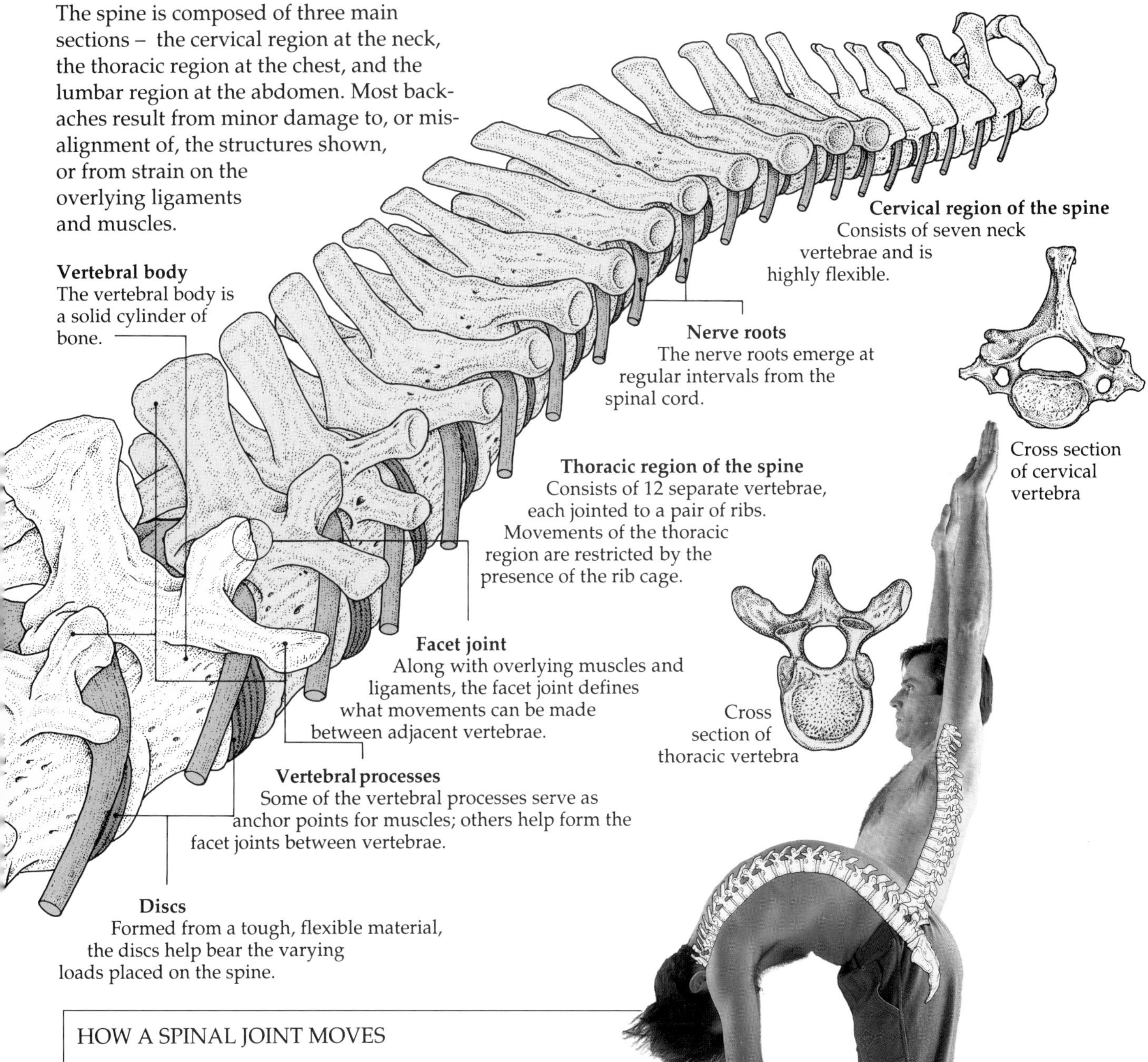

Vertebral body
The vertebral body is a solid cylinder of bone.

Cervical region of the spine
Consists of seven neck vertebrae and is highly flexible.

Nerve roots
The nerve roots emerge at regular intervals from the spinal cord.

Thoracic region of the spine
Consists of 12 separate vertebrae, each jointed to a pair of ribs. Movements of the thoracic region are restricted by the presence of the rib cage.

Cross section of cervical vertebra

Facet joint
Along with overlying muscles and ligaments, the facet joint defines what movements can be made between adjacent vertebrae.

Cross section of thoracic vertebra

Vertebral processes
Some of the vertebral processes serve as anchor points for muscles; others help form the facet joints between vertebrae.

Discs
Formed from a tough, flexible material, the discs help bear the varying loads placed on the spine.

HOW A SPINAL JOINT MOVES

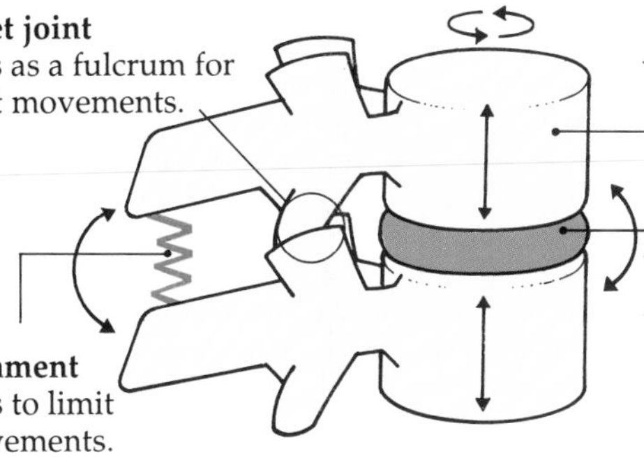

Facet joint
Acts as a fulcrum for joint movements.

Vertebral body

Ligament
Acts to limit movements.

Disc
Acts as a shock absorber and also like a ball bearing, allowing a variety of joint movements.

Spinal movements and stresses
The range of movement of individual spinal joints is relatively small, but in combination they give the spine a wide range of movement. When bending forward or backward, most of the movement is in the lower back. If movement takes place against strong resistance (as when lifting a heavy object), great stress is created, which can easily lead to minor damage of the muscles, ligaments, or discs, with consequent pain in the lumbar region.

Back pain occurs most often in the lower back – the region of the lumbar vertebrae. Although this part of the back bears the greatest load, its structure is also capable of a wide range of bending, side-to-side, and twisting movements. Consequently, great stress is placed on each of its components. Unless care is taken with posture and movement, a relatively minor incident may trigger an injury. As is the case with so many of our body systems, prevention is the key to avoiding back disorders.

ACUTE BACK PAIN

Acute back pain can develop over a relatively short period of time, which is what occurs with most low back pain. Back pain that develops gradually over time is more likely to persist and become chronic, meaning that the pain is long-standing and tends to recur.

Who is at risk?

Back pain most commonly affects those between the ages of 30 and 60. Few people under 18 and over 60 are affected by back problems. In part, these statistics reflect the greater demands placed on adults during their working years. However, it is also true that teenagers have flexible backs and that in the elderly the spine becomes less flexible, which protects it against many kinds of strain by limiting the older person's range of motion.

You are more likely to experience back pain if your daily activities involve lifting and carrying. If you are not accustomed to heavy work it is important to be careful when you do it (see HOW TO PREVENT BACK PAIN on pages 70 and 71).

Working in a cramped space in an awkward or bent-over position may also cause back pain. In addition, people with sedentary jobs are at high risk of developing back pain, particularly if they sit in one position for long periods. Truck drivers and airplane pilots, for example, tend to experience low back pain.

THREE COMMON CAUSES OF BACK PAIN

Back pain has a wide range of possible causes. However, many of the people in whom acute back pain develops suddenly can attribute their pain to one of the causes shown below. All can be classified as mechanical causes of back pain – none involve any serious underlying disease. With each of these causes, the pain usually eases after resting for between 24 hours and a week.

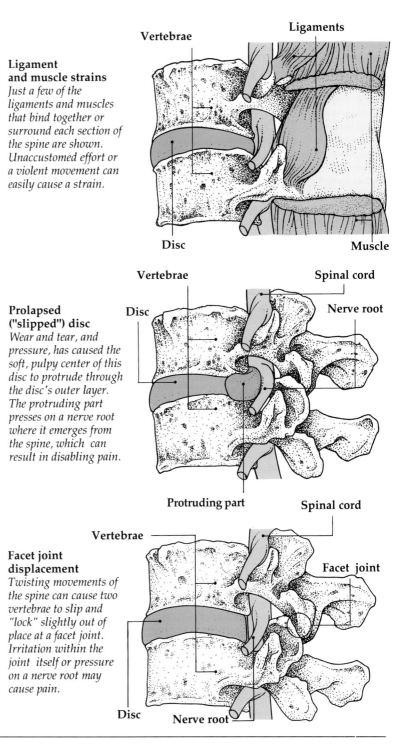

Ligament and muscle strains
Just a few of the ligaments and muscles that bind together or surround each section of the spine are shown. Unaccustomed effort or a violent movement can easily cause a strain.

Vertebrae — Ligaments — Disc — Muscle

Prolapsed ("slipped") disc
Wear and tear, and pressure, has caused the soft, pulpy center of this disc to protrude through the disc's outer layer. The protruding part presses on a nerve root where it emerges from the spine, which can result in disabling pain.

Vertebrae — Spinal cord — Disc — Nerve root — Protruding part

Facet joint displacement
Twisting movements of the spine can cause two vertebrae to slip and "lock" slightly out of place at a facet joint. Irritation within the joint itself or pressure on a nerve root may cause pain.

Vertebrae — Spinal cord — Facet joint — Disc — Nerve root

CASE HISTORY
LOW BACK PAIN

Gᴇᴏʀɢᴇ's ʙᴀᴄᴋ ᴘᴀɪɴ **started 2 days after moving some furniture into his new apartment. He awoke with severe pain and stiffness in his lower back. Deciding that he must have strained his back, he took some aspirin. However, after resting for 3 days he felt no better, so he called his doctor.**

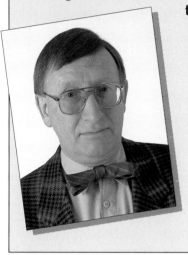

PERSONAL DETAILS
Name George Clark
Age 57
Occupation Copywriter for an advertising agency
Family Father has suffered repeated episodes of back strain. Mother is well.

MEDICAL BACKGROUND
George hasn't seen a doctor for more than 10 years. He has suffered twinges of pain in his back but it has never kept him home from work.

THE CONSULTATION
George describes the pain in his back. The pain is getting worse and has spread into his right buttock and down the back of his right thigh.

On examination, the doctor finds that George is unable to stand up straight. The muscles over the right side of his back are in spasm (contracted and unable to relax) and his spine is tilted to the right. He cannot touch his knees and all movements of his spine are painful.

George is helped up onto the examination table where he lies flat on his back. The doctor lifts each leg with the knee kept straight. The left leg can be raised to a right angle with the table, but the right leg can be lifted to an angle of only 30 degrees. The doctor then checks the power, sensation, and reflexes in George's legs. He finds no sign of damage to the spinal nerves.

THE DOCTOR'S IMPRESSION
The doctor suspects a diagnosis of a ᴘʀᴏʟᴀᴘꜱᴇᴅ ᴅɪꜱᴄ ("slipped," or herniated, disc) in George's lower back. His findings indicate that part of one of the discs between two of George s vertebrae is protruding and pressing on one of the right lumbar nerve roots at the point where it emerges from the spine. This accounts for the pain (sciatica) in George's right leg and buttock. It also accounts for the difficulty in raising his right leg on the examination table. However, the doctor decides that George does not require a spinal X-ray.

THE TREATMENT
George is advised to rest at home on a flat surface and is given a prescription for some painkillers and a muscle relaxant to ease the spasm in his back. A week later, the movements of George's spine are still restricted and the doctor finds George is unable to raise his right leg more than 70 degrees above the examination table. George is advised to rest another week at home, and then make an appointment with a physical therapist. An X-ray is scheduled to rule out any abnormality in the bones and joints.

By the time George sees the therapist, his back is free of pain and he has regained a full range of movement. He is given an exercise program to strengthen his abdominal and spinal muscles and is advised to lose at least 10 pounds to reduce the strain on his lower back.

THE OUTCOME
The X-rays show signs of osteoarthritis in George's lower spine. However, since he has recovered , it appears that the back pain has been caused by the disc prolapse, not by the arthritis. George resolves to take more care in the future when moving heavy objects.

The physical examination
The difficulty in raising George's right leg above an angle of 30 degrees on the examination table is a clue to the diagnosis.

MONITOR YOUR SYMPTOMS
PAINFUL BACK

Occasional mild back pain is common and is usually a sign of slight damage or strain. Severe pain may have a more serious cause. Persistent back pain is much less common; inflammatory and degenerative conditions affecting the spine are among possible causes. Any severe or persistent back pain requires medical attention.

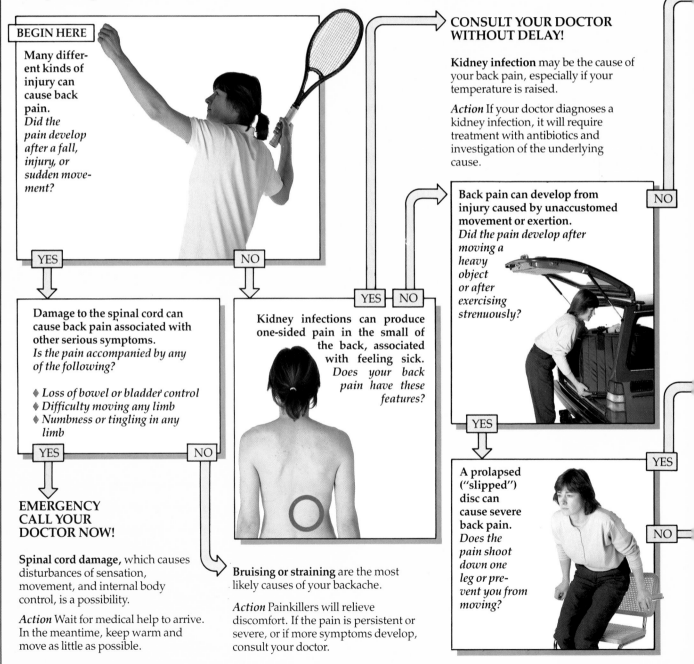

WARNING

Whatever the history and pattern of your back pain, consult a doctor immediately if you also suffer any loss of bowel or bladder control, or weakness, numbness, or tingling in an arm or leg.

BEGIN HERE

Many different kinds of injury can cause back pain.
Did the pain develop after a fall, injury, or sudden movement?

YES   NO

CONSULT YOUR DOCTOR WITHOUT DELAY!

Kidney infection may be the cause of your back pain, especially if your temperature is raised.

Action If your doctor diagnoses a kidney infection, it will require treatment with antibiotics and investigation of the underlying cause.

Back pain can develop from injury caused by unaccustomed movement or exertion.
Did the pain develop after moving a heavy object or after exercising strenuously?

NO

YES   NO

Damage to the spinal cord can cause back pain associated with other serious symptoms.
Is the pain accompanied by any of the following?

♦ *Loss of bowel or bladder control*
♦ *Difficulty moving any limb*
♦ *Numbness or tingling in any limb*

YES   NO

Kidney infections can produce one-sided pain in the small of the back, associated with feeling sick.
Does your back pain have these features?

YES

A prolapsed ("slipped") disc can cause severe back pain.
Does the pain shoot down one leg or prevent you from moving?

YES

NO

EMERGENCY CALL YOUR DOCTOR NOW!

Spinal cord damage, which causes disturbances of sensation, movement, and internal body control, is a possibility.

Action Wait for medical help to arrive. In the meantime, keep warm and move as little as possible.

Bruising or straining are the most likely causes of your backache.

Action Painkillers will relieve discomfort. If the pain is persistent or severe, or if more symptoms develop, consult your doctor.

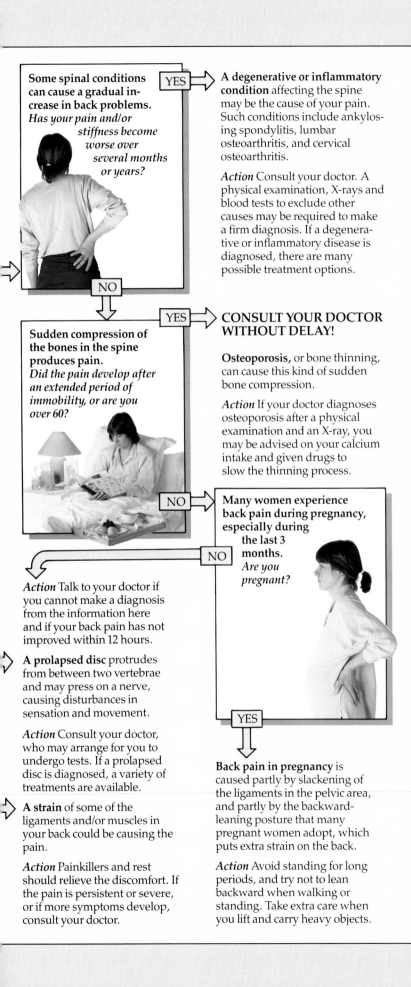

Some spinal conditions can cause a gradual increase in back problems. *Has your pain and/or stiffness become worse over several months or years?*

YES

A degenerative or inflammatory condition affecting the spine may be the cause of your pain. Such conditions include ankylosing spondylitis, lumbar osteoarthritis, and cervical osteoarthritis.

Action Consult your doctor. A physical examination, X-rays and blood tests to exclude other causes may be required to make a firm diagnosis. If a degenerative or inflammatory disease is diagnosed, there are many possible treatment options.

NO

YES

CONSULT YOUR DOCTOR WITHOUT DELAY!

Osteoporosis, or bone thinning, can cause this kind of sudden bone compression.

Action If your doctor diagnoses osteoporosis after a physical examination and an X-ray, you may be advised on your calcium intake and given drugs to slow the thinning process.

Sudden compression of the bones in the spine produces pain. *Did the pain develop after an extended period of immobility, or are you over 60?*

NO

Many women experience back pain during pregnancy, especially during the last 3 months. *Are you pregnant?*

NO

Action Talk to your doctor if you cannot make a diagnosis from the information here and if your back pain has not improved within 12 hours.

A prolapsed disc protrudes from between two vertebrae and may press on a nerve, causing disturbances in sensation and movement.

Action Consult your doctor, who may arrange for you to undergo tests. If a prolapsed disc is diagnosed, a variety of treatments are available.

A strain of some of the ligaments and/or muscles in your back could be causing the pain.

Action Painkillers and rest should relieve the discomfort. If the pain is persistent or severe, or if more symptoms develop, consult your doctor.

YES

Back pain in pregnancy is caused partly by slackening of the ligaments in the pelvic area, and partly by the backward-leaning posture that many pregnant women adopt, which puts extra strain on the back.

Action Avoid standing for long periods, and try not to lean backward when walking or standing. Take extra care when you lift and carry heavy objects.

You are also more at risk of back pain if you are overweight, because your back is carrying a heavier load, the abdominal muscles that help support your spine may be weak, and the extra weight often contributes to poor posture.

What are the causes?

In many cases, acute back pain is simply a normal reaction to unaccustomed use. If you don't exercise often and then spend a day moving furniture or digging in the garden, you should expect some pain in your lower back as the day goes on. The following day, your back may be stiff and painful. This is normal; the pain and stiffness are due to a passing spasm in the muscles and a mild strain of the ligaments in your back.

In some cases, there may be minor damage to, or a strain of, one of the back's ligaments or muscles. This can occur through overstretching or through lifting a heavy weight awkwardly. You may feel a sudden, sharp pain in your back or may even feel something "go." You should regard this as a clear warning to stop lifting or stretching, but usually the damage is not serious. Afterward, a tender spot can often be found among the muscles of your lower back.

Ligament and muscle strains are examples of nonspecific back pain – so called because tests such as X-rays show nothing wrong. Usually, with rest and the use of painkillers, the pain disappears before extensive tests are needed.

Other common causes of sudden back pain are facet joint displacements and disc prolapses (commonly called "slipped" discs, though this is a misnomer since discs cannot slip out of position). These injuries tend to cause more severe and persistent pain. In a facet joint displacement, which often follows a twisting movement, two or more adjacent spinal vertebrae move slightly out of alignment. With a disc prolapse, part of the tough outer layer of the disc between two vertebrae ruptures, allowing the soft center of the disc to protrude outward. The protrusion puts pressure on one of the nerves that emerge from the spine. A disc prolapse can result from a minor injury if the disc has been weakened by previous wear and tear.

With both facet joint displacements and disc prolapse, muscles overlying the affected joint tend to go into spasm, which can make the pain worse. A disc prolapse may also cause shooting pains down one leg (called sciatica). Coughing, laughing, or straining to move the bowels may increase the pain.

What can be done?

Most acute back pain subsides if the damaged part of the spine is given time to heal. It is often helped by resting for a minimum of 24 hours on a firm mattress or board, or by lying flat on a hard surface such as the floor. For most people, bed rest is required for a longer period.

Try to avoid any position or movement that aggravates the pain. If you have to sit, make sure that you sit up straight, well back in the chair. When you get up from sitting or lying, push up with your arms to reduce the stress on your spine. To move from a lying position, roll to the edge of the bed and lower your legs to the floor at the same time you raise your upper body.

To ease the pain, take aspirin or acetaminophen. You can also apply heat with a heating pad or hot-water bottle.

PERSISTENT BACK PAIN

If back pain is persistent and does not respond to home treatment within a week, consult your doctor, who may want to perform some tests. A spinal X-ray may be used to reveal any bone or joint abnormality such as osteoarthritis of the spine, ankylosing spondylitis (inflammation of the spinal joints), a stress fracture of a vertebra, a spondylolisthesis (forward displacement of a vertebra), or even bone cancer. However, an X-ray does not show any damage to a ligament, muscle, facet joint, or disc. Your

HOW TO PREVENT BACK PAIN

Many back injuries are caused by putting the muscles of the back under too much strain. Paying attention to your posture and avoiding certain awkward movements can reduce the risk of straining and injuring your back.

Sitting
Find a chair with a firm, upright back that supports the spine. The chair should be of a size and height that enables you to place your feet flat on the ground and to bend your knees comfortably at a right angle. The seat should support most of the back of your thighs.

Lifting a heavy load
Moving a heavy object places a great deal of strain on the spine. To avoid injury, bend your knees and keep your lower back straight. Don't reach forward or to one side as you lift; make sure the object is directly in front of you and not too far away (figure 1). Return to a standing position by pushing up from your knees and keeping the back straight, as shown in figures 2, 3, and 4.

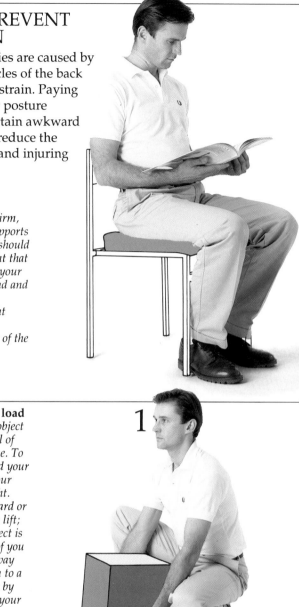

doctor may recommend more tests to examine these areas in detail.

The treatment of persistent back pain depends on the cause. If there is a mechanical problem that has not improved with rest, traction or injections of anti-inflammatory drugs may be helpful.

Only about 2 percent of back pain cases are treated by surgery. A prolapsed disc that has caused intense pain for a long period can be treated surgically.

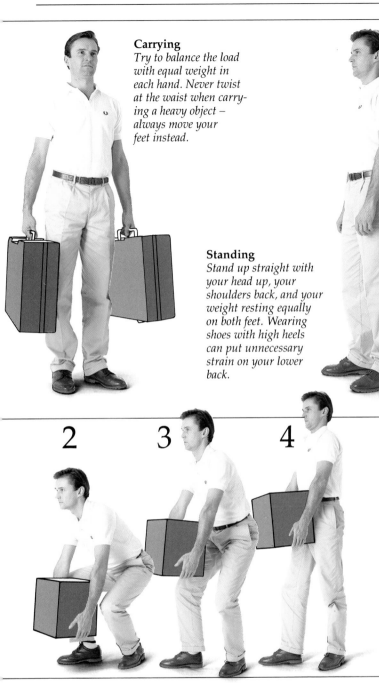

Carrying
Try to balance the load with equal weight in each hand. Never twist at the waist when carrying a heavy object – always move your feet instead.

Standing
Stand up straight with your head up, your shoulders back, and your weight resting equally on both feet. Wearing shoes with high heels can put unnecessary strain on your lower back.

In rare cases, people who have a permanent displacement of one of the vertebrae, or severe osteoarthritis, may have an operation in which adjacent vertebrae are strengthened by being bonded together with bone grafts or with metal screws and plates. In addition, surgery is sometimes used to remove a tumor in the spinal cord. Bone cancer is treated by radiation therapy, chemotherapy, and, occasionally, surgery.

ASK YOUR DOCTOR BACK PAIN

Q I have recently been treated with traction for a slipped disc. My back pain is now gone, but will the disc slip again once I go back to work and become more active?

A A slipped disc has not really "slipped." What has happened is that part of the pulpy, inner portion of the disc has protruded through the outer layer of the disc so that it presses on a nearby nerve root emerging from the spinal canal. Traction eases the pain by relieving the pressure, but the protruding part of the disc shrinks back to normal slowly. To reduce the risk of pain recurring, you should exercise to strengthen your back muscles, avoid awkward movements and postures, and take extra care when you lift or carry anything heavy.

Q I have been told that back pain is almost always due to arthritis and won't get better. Is this true?

A It is true that many people have signs of osteoarthritis when their spines are X-rayed and that arthritis is difficult to treat. However, osteoarthritis tends to progress gradually, so it is unlikely to be the cause of any sudden back pain. A muscle or ligament strain is much more likely. Disc prolapse is a less common cause.

Q My teenage daughter insists on wearing high-heeled shoes every day. Is this bad for her back?

A Yes, wearing high heels regularly will alter the alignment of your daughter's body. The lower part of her spine, which bears her weight, will tilt forward, placing pressure on muscles, ligaments, and joints of the lumbar region.

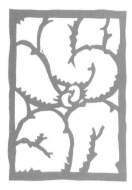

BOWEL AND DIGESTIVE PROBLEMS

BEFORE THE DISCOVERY of X-rays, surgeons called the abdomen the "temple of surprises" because they were never quite sure what they would find inside of it. With the help of modern equipment, doctors today can identify most serious digestive tract problems at an early stage. However, the majority of problems are minor.

The digestive tract consists of a series of specialized conduits and food processing chambers, each with its own functions and disorders. The disorders are described here from the top downward.

SWALLOWING DIFFICULTY AND HEARTBURN

Difficulty swallowing is not common, but it can be distressing and may occasionally have a serious cause. A sore throat may cause discomfort when swallowing, or the difficulty may result from a small foreign object, such as a fish bone or chicken bone, lodged at the back of the throat or in the esophagus.

Discomfort can also be caused by inflammation of, or damage to, the lining of the esophagus. This can occur from eating or drinking something very hot, from a tablet (such as an aspirin tablet) that has become stuck in the esophagus and corroded its lining, or, most common of all, from reflux of acid into the esophagus from the stomach. Acid reflux, known as heartburn, is usually noticed as a burning pain behind the breastbone (see WHAT IS HEARTBURN? on page 62).

Other possible causes of swallowing difficulty include disorders of the esophageal muscles, which help propel food toward the stomach, or, in rare cases, a tumor of the esophagus.

What can be done?

A small foreign object may be dislodged by eating a little dry bread, but you should always see your doctor if you know that you have swallowed something sharp, even if you are not experiencing any discomfort or pain.

Minor damage or inflammation of the esophagus that is causing discomfort usually heals after a day or two. You can prevent a recurrence of the problem by avoiding very hot food or drink, and by washing down any pills you take with a large glass of water.

If you have persistent difficulty swallowing, painful swallowing, or continual regurgitation, see your doctor.

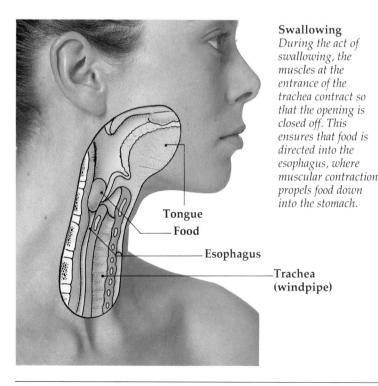

Swallowing
During the act of swallowing, the muscles at the entrance of the trachea contract so that the opening is closed off. This ensures that food is directed into the esophagus, where muscular contraction propels food down into the stomach.

Tongue
Food
Esophagus
Trachea (windpipe)

WHERE DO THE PROBLEMS OCCUR?

Think of the digestive tract as a kind of processing plant that breaks down the components of food for absorption from the intestines into the bloodstream and expels the waste products from the body. A variety of disorders may affect the different parts of the tract, as illustrated below. Some of these disorders disrupt the digestive process, others are a problem mainly because they cause pain or symptoms such as diarrhea.

Pharynx

Esophagus

Liver

Stomach

Colon

Duodenum

Small intestine

Rectum

Gallbladder
Stones may form within this small organ, sometimes causing inflammation and pain.

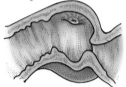

Duodenal ulcer

Duodenum
Painful peptic ulcers may form in the lining of the duodenum.

Colon
Irregular contractions of the walls of the colon may occur, causing diarrhea or constipation. Other disorders include various infections and inflammatory conditions, diverticular disease, and tumors.

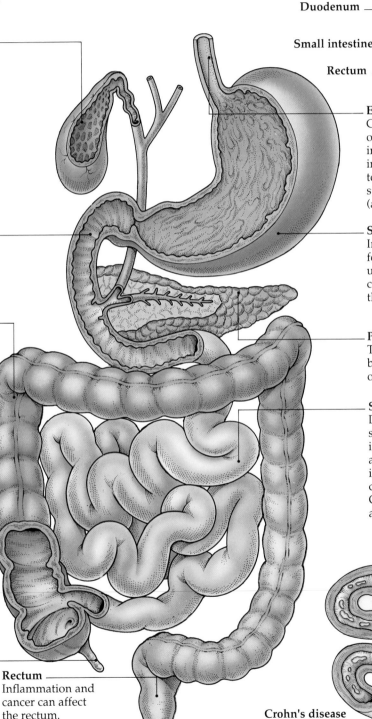

Esophagus
Common disorders of the esophagus include inflammation due to acid reflux and strictures (abnormal narrowing).

Stomach
Indigestion and the formation of peptic ulcers are the most common problems in the stomach.

Pancreas
The pancreas may become acutely or chronically inflamed.

Small intestine
Disorders of the small intestine include failure to absorb nutrients, inflammatory conditions such as Crohn's disease, and infections.

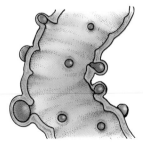

Diverticular disease

Appendix
The appendix may become severely inflamed.

Rectum
Inflammation and cancer can affect the rectum.

Crohn's disease

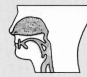

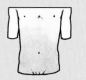
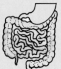
GAS AND INDIGESTION

Indigestion is the common feeling of abdominal pain and bloating after a meal. It is often accompanied by nausea and heartburn. If excess gas is present in the stomach or intestine, it may be expelled from the body through the mouth by belching or through the anus as gas (flatulence).

What are the causes?

Indigestion and gas may be caused by overeating and overdrinking, or by certain foods. Each of us reacts differently to individual foods and, over time, we identify those most likely to cause indigestion or gas. Persistent flatulence is a common symptom of irritable bowel syndrome. One expression of this condition is an abnormally strong and irregular contraction of the muscles that propel waste material through the intestine, resulting in constipation, diarrhea, or alternating bouts of the two.

Rhythmic pain or nausea coming on an hour or two after meals or in the middle of the night can be a symptom of

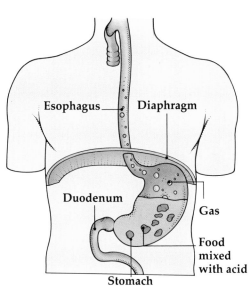

What happens inside the stomach?
Food is mixed with hydrochloric acid and broken down to a liquid consistency in the stomach. Indigestion may result from acid irritating the stomach lining, or from stomach bloating caused by overeating and gas production.

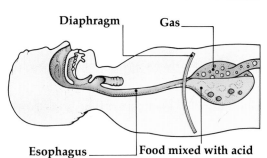

Why do doctors advise against lying down too soon after a meal?
When you lie down, acid may flow back from the stomach into the esophagus and cause pain (heartburn). Gas is also more likely to move into the intestines, causing bloating and discomfort.

ulceration in the lining of the stomach or duodenum. This condition is also called peptic ulcer. The exact cause of peptic ulcers is unknown, but the chances of one developing are increased if you smoke or drink heavily or if you regularly take aspirin or related drugs.

Severe anxiety or nervousness may cause belching because these emotions encourage the swallowing of air. Stress, if prolonged, may contribute to the development of peptic ulcers or to irritable bowel syndrome.

Finally, gallstones (hard deposits) may cause no symptoms or may cause acute inflammation of the gallbladder, pain, and vomiting. Gallstones leaving the gallbladder sometimes block the bile ducts (see pages 76 and 77).

What can be done?

Antacids usually help relieve attacks of mild indigestion. If you suffer from belching or gas, follow some of the self-help measures suggested opposite.

Peptic ulcers respond to antacids or drugs that diminish the secretion of gastric acid. Pain relief and healing usually occur within 6 weeks. Eliminating alcohol from your diet and giving up cigarettes helps the healing process.

Irritable bowel syndrome can usually be improved by an increase in dietary fiber. If symptoms persist, your doctor may prescribe medication to prevent muscle spasm of the colon.

MONITOR YOUR SYMPTOMS
GAS

The presence of excess gas in the digestive system is a common, sometimes embarrassing, symptom, but it is rarely the result of a serious condition. Gas is usually caused by swallowing air or by eating foods that ferment in the intestine.

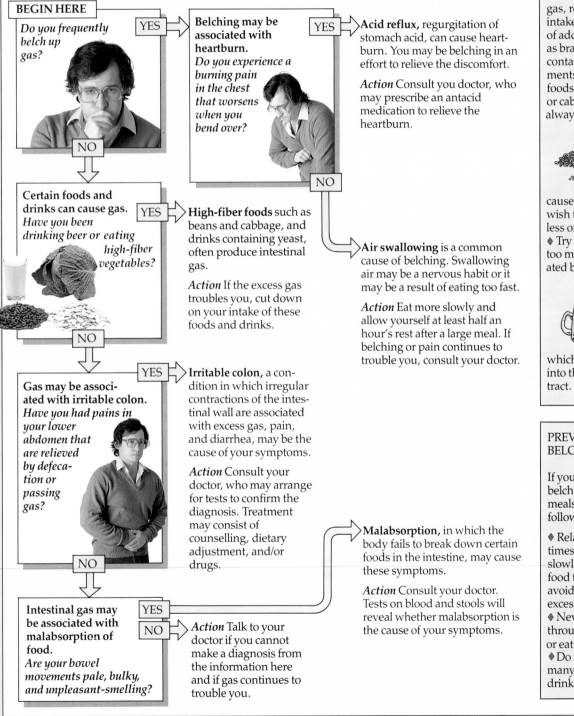

BEGIN HERE

Do you frequently belch up gas? — **YES** →

Belching may be associated with heartburn.
Do you experience a burning pain in the chest that worsens when you bend over? — **YES** →

Acid reflux, regurgitation of stomach acid, can cause heartburn. You may be belching in an effort to relieve the discomfort.

Action Consult you doctor, who may prescribe an antacid medication to relieve the heartburn.

NO ↓

NO ↓

Certain foods and drinks can cause gas.
Have you been drinking beer or eating high-fiber vegetables? — **YES** →

High-fiber foods such as beans and cabbage, and drinks containing yeast, often produce intestinal gas.

Action If the excess gas troubles you, cut down on your intake of these foods and drinks.

Air swallowing is a common cause of belching. Swallowing air may be a nervous habit or it may be a result of eating too fast.

Action Eat more slowly and allow yourself at least half an hour's rest after a large meal. If belching or pain continues to trouble you, consult your doctor.

NO ↓

Gas may be associated with irritable colon.
Have you had pains in your lower abdomen that are relieved by defecation or passing gas? — **YES** →

Irritable colon, a condition in which irregular contractions of the intestinal wall are associated with excess gas, pain, and diarrhea, may be the cause of your symptoms.

Action Consult your doctor, who may arrange for tests to confirm the diagnosis. Treatment may consist of counselling, dietary adjustment, and/or drugs.

Malabsorption, in which the body fails to break down certain foods in the intestine, may cause these symptoms.

Action Consult your doctor. Tests on blood and stools will reveal whether malabsorption is the cause of your symptoms.

NO ↓

Intestinal gas may be associated with malabsorption of food.
Are your bowel movements pale, bulky, and unpleasant-smelling?

YES →

NO →

Action Talk to your doctor if you cannot make a diagnosis from the information here and if gas continues to trouble you.

HOW TO PREVENT INTESTINAL GAS

The following self-help measures may improve a problem with excess gas:

♦ If a sudden increase in dietary fiber has caused gas, reduce your intake, particularly of added fiber such as bran or fiber-containing supplements. If certain foods, such as beans or cabbage, always

cause gas, you may wish to eat them less often.
♦ Try not to drink too many carbonated beverages,

which introduce gas into the digestive tract.

PREVENTING BELCHING

If you frequently belch up gas after meals, try the following:

♦ Relax at mealtimes. Always eat slowly and chew food thoroughly to avoid swallowing excess air.
♦ Never rush through your meals or eat while standing.
♦ Do not drink too many carbonated drinks.

ABDOMINAL PAIN

At one time or another, everyone experiences minor abdominal pain, which may be accompanied by gas, constipation, or diarrhea. Only occasionally is such pain a symptom of a serious disorder.

What are the causes?

If abdominal pain follows a period of overeating or overdrinking, the cause may be easily recognized. However, there are many other possible causes of such pain. Many women experience cramping abdominal pain at the time of their menstrual period. While this pain is uncomfortable, it is not usually serious. However, severe pain may indicate a disorder of the uterus, ovaries, or fallopian tubes and should be investigated by your doctor. Cystitis (inflammation of the bladder) is another common cause of lower abdominal pain, especially in women (see page 84).

Gastroenteritis (inflammation of the stomach and intestinal lining) causes periodic waves of abdominal pain, known as colic, as the muscles of the intestine go into spasm. Colicky pain may also be a

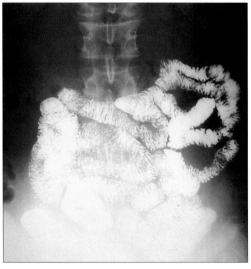

The small intestine
The X-ray image above shows how the small intestine is coiled up to fit inside the abdominal cavity. Spasms in the muscular wall of the intestine may be a cause of bouts of abdominal pain.

symptom of cholecystitis, an inflammation of the gallbladder caused by a stone blocking a bile duct. Renal colic is a severe pain in the lower back caused by the passing of a kidney stone down a ureter toward the bladder.

Severe pain and tenderness with vomiting and fever suggest an acute inflammation of one of the organs in the abdominal cavity. Peritonitis (inflammation of the membrane that lines the abdominal cavity) may result from acute appendicitis, cholecystitis, salpingitis (inflammation of the fallopian tubes), diverticular disease (a disorder of the colon), or a perforated peptic ulcer.

HELPLINE
ABDOMINAL PAIN

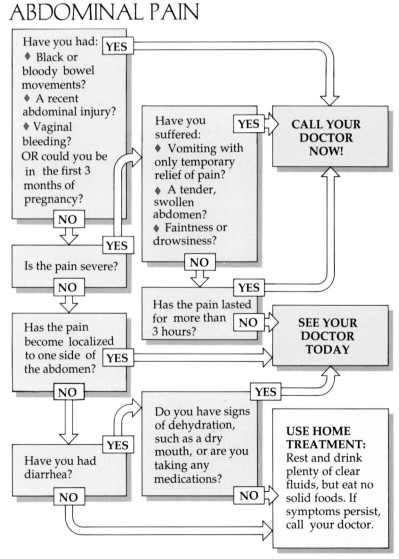

`1 INCH`

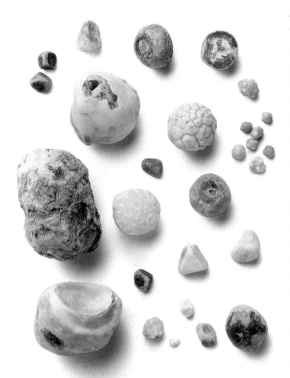

Gallstones
Gallstones differ in appearance and composition depending on whether they contain bile pigment, cholesterol, calcium, or a mixture of all three (see above). Stones may be as small as a grain of sand or as large as a walnut. The color-enhanced X-ray (left) shows the outline of a gallbladder containing gallstones.

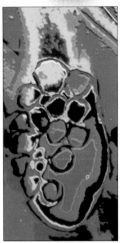

Treating abdominal pain

Simple remedies such as drinking a glass of milk, taking an antacid, or holding a hot-water bottle against the painful area may successfully relieve mild abdominal pain. If these measures are not effective, the cause of the pain should be investigated by a doctor.

The diagnosis of acute abdominal pain can be difficult but should be made quickly. If tests fail to reveal the cause, exploratory surgery may be necessary.

DIARRHEA AND VOMITING

When infectious agents enter the digestive system, the body reacts by emptying the contents of the stomach via the vomiting mechanism and the contents of the intestines through diarrhea. Although these symptoms can occur separately, they are frequently experienced together.

Why do they occur?

The most common cause of diarrhea and vomiting is an infection of the digestive tract, which leads to inflammation and is called gastroenteritis. Gastroenteritis may be the result of eating food contaminated by bacteria or viruses (food poisoning) or may result from a viral infection caught from another person. Such infections may last for anywhere between 2 hours and 3 days and may be accompanied by abdominal pain, fever, aching and weakness.

Diarrhea, nausea, and vomiting can also be caused by antibiotic drugs that can destroy the harmless bacteria in the digestive tract that are needed for successful digestion. If you have persistent diarrhea in the morning, you should be checked by your doctor.

Vomiting on its own can have a variety of causes, including a high temperature in children, motion sickness, a side effect of drugs, or excess alcohol or other ingested contaminants or poisons. If the vomiting is due to a disease of the stomach or intestines, other, more prominent, symptoms are usually present.

Treatment

If you suffer an attack of food poisoning or gastroenteritis, rest quietly at home and drink oral rehydration solution (see right) in frequent, small quantities. When your symptoms begin to improve, you can gradually start eating bland, soft food. Avoid antidiarrheal drugs because they may slow down the elimination of infectious organisms from the body.

Preventing dehydration
Give your child plenty of fluids if he or she is vomiting or having diarrhea.

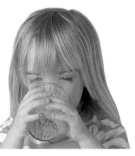

WARNING

Babies, children, and elderly people suffering from diarrhea and vomiting are at particular risk of dehydration from the continuing fluid losses. They should be given 2 to 3 pints of oral rehydration solution per day. You can prepare the solution by adding a premixed packet of ingredients to water, or you can make the solution at home by adding half a teaspoon of salt, 2 teaspoons of sugar, and a quarter of a teaspoon of sodium bicarbonate (baking soda) to 1 pint of water.

Consult your doctor if the child is under 2, if diarrhea and vomiting persist for more than 48 hours, or if signs of dehydration, such as drowsiness, sunken eyes, and dry skin, occur.

CASE HISTORY
GASTROENTERITIS

Peter woke in the early morning with severe, cramping abdominal pains. He was soon violently sick and his bowel movements became loose and frequent. He blamed this on the chili dogs he had eaten the night before. At 8:30 AM Peter telephoned his school to say that he would not be coming in. He was told that several other teachers were suffering from the same symptoms. Peter decided to call his doctor.

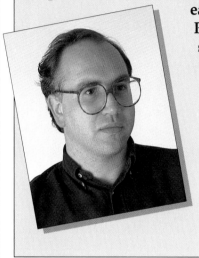

PERSONAL DETAILS
Name Peter Drewbaker
Age 37
Occupation Physics teacher
Family Father had an operation for a duodenal ulcer. Mother is healthy.

MEDICAL BACKGROUND

Peter has had an operation to drain fluid from his middle ears at age 4 and several episodes of tonsillitis as a child. He has had desensitization injections to control symptoms of a pollen allergy for the last 2 years. Otherwise, his general health is good.

THE CONSULTATION

Peter feels too weak to travel to his doctor's office alone, so his neighbor agrees to drive him.

Peter describes his illness, which he thinks might be due to the chili dogs, but he also mentions that some of his colleagues at work had devel-

oped the same symptoms overnight. He seems worried about a possible epidemic at the school. He says that, during the night, he had begun to sweat and had felt chilled. His bowel movements became very loose, almost like water, and each movement was preceded by brief spasms of abdominal pain. Two teaspoonfuls of an antacid had done little to relieve the discomfort. He still feels nauseated and feverish and has some abdominal discomfort, but he has not vomited for several hours and has not needed to move his bowels for the last hour.

The doctor is interested in the fact that other members of Peter's school are ill and asks him what he has eaten over the previous 2 days, especially food that his colleagues might have shared with him. At first, Peter does not think shared food could be responsible for the illness, but then he remembers that he and a group of other teachers had eaten a chicken, rice, and vegetable casserole served for lunch in the school's staff cafeteria yesterday.

The doctor examines Peter and finds he has a mild fever. He looks dehydrated and has tenderness over his abdomen. His pulse is a little fast and his blood pressure is slightly lower than normal. The doctor gives Peter a container and disposable spatula to collect a small sample of feces for laboratory testing. The doctor has the container delivered to the microbiology department at the hospital the same day.

THE DOCTOR'S IMPRESSION

Peter is likely to be suffering from food poisoning. This condition is generally caused by food contaminated with bacteria, bacterial toxins, or viruses, which lead to an infection of the intestines. The body's reaction is to pour fluid into the intestines,

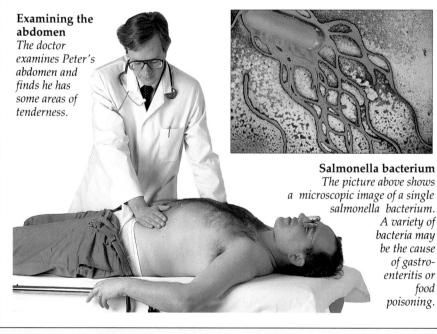

Examining the abdomen
The doctor examines Peter's abdomen and finds he has some areas of tenderness.

Salmonella bacterium
The picture above shows a microscopic image of a single salmonella bacterium. A variety of bacteria may be the cause of gastroenteritis or food poisoning.

which results in diarrhea. The infection also causes a fever, and toxins produced by the bacteria are involved in triggering the nausea and vomiting. The infection also accounts for Peter's raised pulse and lowered blood pressure. And because the same symptoms have developed in several other people simultaneously, the doctor believes a specific food was to blame.

THE DIAGNOSIS

The results of the laboratory tests on Peter's feces and those of his colleagues confirm the doctor's diagnosis of SALMONELLA FOOD POISONING.

THE TREATMENT

Peter is not ill enough to be admitted to the hospital; he is no longer vomiting, and his abdominal pain and diarrhea have eased. He is given an oral electrolyte mixture to drink to replace the body fluids lost through vomiting and diarrhea. He is advised to drink uncarbonated, clear fluids but not to eat any food for at least 24 hours. He is not allowed to drink alcohol, which could cause more dehydration. Once the diarrhea has stopped for several hours, Peter can eat again, starting with soup, bread, cereal, and eggs.

THE OUTCOME

Peter made a rapid recovery and was soon able to return to school. The outbreak of food poisoning prompted a visit to the school's staff cafeteria by a health officer, who found several unsatisfactory cooking and storage practices. Cooked and raw meat were stored side by side in the refrigerator, and salads were prepared on the same surface as raw meat without adequate cleaning in between. Steps were taken immediately to improve hygiene in the school's kitchen.

HOW TO PREVENT FOOD POISONING

Common sources of food poisoning include poultry; seafood; meat that is undercooked, inadequately defrosted, or reheated; and raw or lightly cooked eggs. Food poisoning can usually be avoided by following the precautions suggested below:

YOU SHOULD:

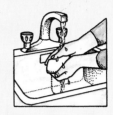

♦ Always wash your hands before handling food and after handling raw meat.

♦ Clean utensils and cutting boards thoroughly with soap and very hot water after preparing raw meat.

♦ Wash fresh fruit and vegetables in cold, running water.

♦ Allow meat and poultry to thaw completely before cooking. Thawing is best done in a microwave oven or in a refrigerator, where the food may be kept for 24 hours after thawing. Meat that has thawed in the refrigerator should be cooked soon after thawing.

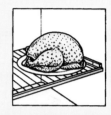

♦ Store fresh fish in the freezer and wash it thoroughly before cooking.

♦ Keep egg dishes in the refrigerator.

♦ Take care to sterilize food thoroughly when you preserve it at home by heating it in a pressure cooker at 250°F (120°C) for 30 minutes.

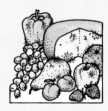

♦ Reheat meat quickly and thoroughly.

♦ Make sure that gravy made from meat fat or juices is heated thoroughly and served hot.

♦ Eat meat as soon as it has been cooked.

♦ Cover up cooked meat and put leftover cooked meat in the refrigerator once it has cooled and within 90 minutes.

♦ Discard food that has become moldy or smelly and throw away any damaged or bulging cans.

YOU SHOULD NOT:

♦ Handle food if you have a sore throat, infected eye, bad cold, upset stomach, or infected cut or sore on your hand.

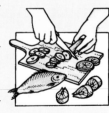

♦ Prepare meat on the same surface as vegetables or cooked meat, or use the same utensils without first washing them with soap and hot water.

♦ Allow egg dishes or creamy foods to stand in a warm kitchen or eat them after they have been at room temperature for more than several hours.

♦ Eat food that looks or smells suspicious or has been kept (even in a refrigerator) too long.

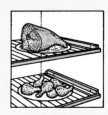

♦ Store raw meat where it may come into contact with cooked meat, or allow water or blood from raw meat to drip onto other food during preparation or storage.

CONSTIPATION

Constipation is rarely a symptom of a serious disorder, but it can lead to anal problems due to straining during defecation. The normal frequency of bowel movements varies greatly. Some people need to empty their bowels two to three times a day, others only once or twice a week. Lack of daily movement is no cause for concern, providing the bowel movement is not hard, dry, and difficult to pass. However, a sudden, persistent change in your normal bowel habits needs investigation by your doctor.

What causes constipation?

Lack of sufficient fiber in the diet is the most common cause of constipation. Some people become constipated by ignoring the urge to defecate. When the urge occurs, they feel they are too busy with other activities to spend time in the bathroom. Constipation eventually occurs because the normal urge to move the bowels is lost. More water is then absorbed into the wall of the colon from the stool, which becomes hard and dry and more difficult to pass.

Many medicines, including iron supplements and painkillers, can cause constipation. The frequent use of laxatives can increase constipation because the sluggish colon becomes dependent upon them for regular movement.

Treating constipation

If you think a poor diet is causing constipation, try to increase the amount of fluids and fiber-containing foods in your diet, including whole-grain cereals and fruits and vegetables (see FIGHTING DIGESTIVE PROBLEMS WITH FIBER above right). If constipation persists for more than 2 weeks, seek medical advice. A serious problem is unlikely but, infrequently, the onset of constipation may indicate an underlying disease such as cancer of the colon. Early examination and treatment is likely to be curative.

FIGHTING DIGESTIVE PROBLEMS WITH FIBER

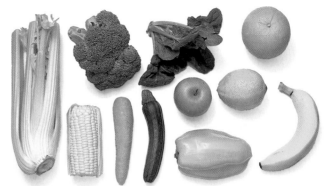

Fibrous roughage – contained in foods such as fresh and dried fruits, whole-grain cereals, raw and green leafy vegetables, nuts, and dried beans – helps prevent digestive problems. The recommended daily intake of fiber is 30 grams. Examples of the quantities of different foods containing this amount are shown below. It is wise, however, to obtain the fiber you need from several different food sources rather than from one source alone.

FOODS CONTAINING 30 GRAMS OF FIBER

9 oz peas (1 cup)

2.4 oz bran (1 cup)

4.5 oz dried apricots (1 cup)

12.6 oz whole-grain bread (10 slices)

11.8 oz Brazil nuts (3 cups)

ANAL PROBLEMS

The anus and the surrounding skin are highly sensitive, but most problems can be prevented by regular toilet habits, avoiding constipation, and keeping the area clean.

When do problems occur?

Hemorrhoids are very common and are usually caused by straining to defecate.

Two less common anal problems are anal fissures and anal abscesses. Anal fissures may cause blood on the toilet paper and painful defecation. Many

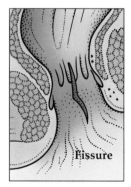

Anal fissure
An anal fissure is a painful crack in the wall of the anal canal that sometimes develops after passing very hard feces.

people, particularly children and the elderly, suffer from itching around the anus, known as pruritus ani. It can be caused by hemorrhoids, anal fissures, thrush, and some sexually transmitted diseases, but sometimes it is simply the result of skin sensitivity. Pinworms are another common cause of anal itching, especially in children.

Treating anal problems

Anyone suffering from hemorrhoids should try not to strain during defecation; it is also important to avoid constipation. Over-the-counter ointments can help ease the pain and irritation of hemorrhoids or pruritus ani. Taking a sitz bath (after a bowel movement, if possible) a couple of times a day will help reduce hemorrhoidal swelling. Persistent hemorrhoids, or any other persistent anal problem, should be brought to the attention of your doctor, as should recurrent itching in a child. Recurrent itching in children may be due to a pinworm infection, which is easily diagnosed and cleared up with drugs.

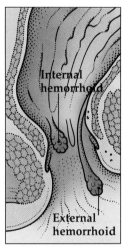

Hemorrhoids
Hemorrhoids are swollen, varicose veins that may develop inside the wall of the anal canal (internal hemorrhoids) or may protrude from the anal opening (external hemorrhoids).

THE STRUCTURE OF THE ANUS

The anus is normally kept tightly closed by the internal and external sphincter muscles, which relax to allow defecation.

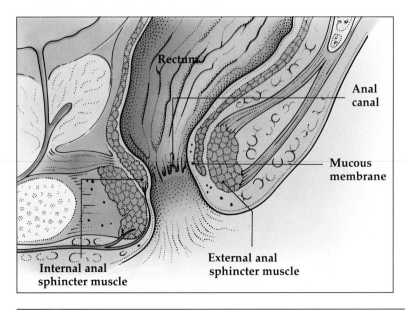

Rectum

Anal canal

Mucous membrane

Internal anal sphincter muscle

External anal sphincter muscle

ASK YOUR DOCTOR
BOWEL AND DIGESTIVE PROBLEMS

Q **My husband has a large swelling on the middle of his abdomen, which he has been told is a hernia. Is it dangerous?**

A Your husband's swelling sounds like a ventral hernia caused by weakness or straining of the muscles of the central abdominal wall. A hernia occasionally becomes dangerous if its blood supply is obstructed. This is something to discuss with your doctor, who may recommend surgery or an abdominal binder.

Q **Since I've been pregnant I've become very constipated. Is there anything I can take for it that won't harm the baby?**

A Constipation is common in pregnancy. Your doctor may prescribe a medicine to soften your feces, but don't take any medication without his or her advice; laxatives should be avoided. A much better approach is to prevent constipation. Eat four to six prunes every day and eat plenty of fruits and vegetables, have some bran or oatmeal, drink eight glasses of water a day, and empty your bowels as soon as you feel the need to.

Q **I've had several attacks of painful diarrhea, with slimy, bloody stools. Could this be cancer?**

A Blood in the stools is something that you should report to your doctor immediately. A severe infection of the digestive tract may be the cause. However, if you have had previous attacks, the cause may be a condition called ulcerative colitis, in which there are raw, inflamed areas along the lining of the intestine.

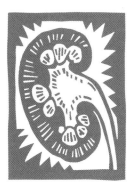

URINARY AND GENITAL PROBLEMS

DISORDERS AFFECTING the urinary tract and the genitals are extremely common. As many as four out of five women suffer from cystitis at some time in their lives. Although the symptoms that can appear in this part of the body are few, the causes are many, so it is wise to consult your doctor for treatment.

The urinary tract is the system that removes waste chemicals and excess water from the body. It consists of the kidneys, ureters, bladder, and urethra. The urinary tract is similar in men and women except that the male urethra is much longer, extending from the base of the bladder to the tip of the penis.

If you are embarrassed by symptoms appearing in this part of your body, remember that urinary and genital problems are very common and your doctor is used to talking about them and finding effective treatment for them.

HOW THE URINARY TRACT WORKS

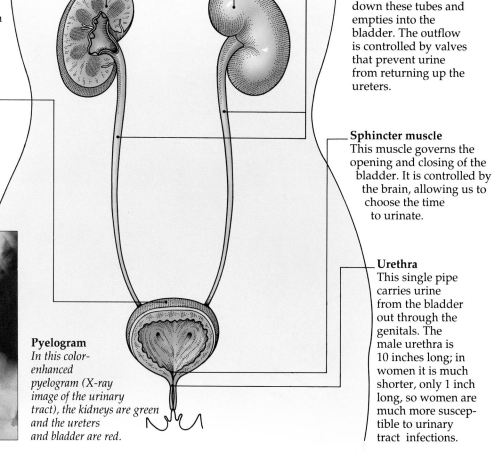

Kidneys
The kidneys remove waste chemicals and water from the blood that passes through them. The water and chemicals, in the form of urine, drain out of the two kidneys via the ureters.

Bladder
The bladder is a temporary storage tank for urine. It has flexible walls, allowing it to expand as it fills; as the bladder reaches capacity, we sense this as the need to urinate. When the bladder empties, its walls contract, forcing the urine out.

Ureters
The urine travels down these tubes and empties into the bladder. The outflow is controlled by valves that prevent urine from returning up the ureters.

Sphincter muscle
This muscle governs the opening and closing of the bladder. It is controlled by the brain, allowing us to choose the time to urinate.

Urethra
This single pipe carries urine from the bladder out through the genitals. The male urethra is 10 inches long; in women it is much shorter, only 1 inch long, so women are much more susceptible to urinary tract infections.

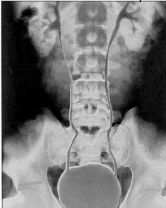

Pyelogram
In this color-enhanced pyelogram (X-ray image of the urinary tract), the kidneys are green and the ureters and bladder are red.

URINARY PROBLEMS

The health problems that affect the urinary tract differ between men and women, both in the symptoms that are suffered and in the underlying causes.

Discomfort during urination

If you feel a painful, burning sensation when passing urine, bacterial infection is the most likely cause. In women, cystitis is the most common culprit (see HOW TO PREVENT CYSTITIS on page 84); otherwise, the pain may be due to a vaginal or urethral infection. Sometimes, bacteria travel up the ureters to the kidneys, causing pain in the back or flank. In men, pain during urination is almost always caused by urethritis, an infection of the urethra that is usually contracted through sexual intercourse.

Frequent urination

The most common cause of an increase in the amount of urine you pass is that you have drunk something, such as coffee, alcohol, or large amounts of water, that increases the blood volume flowing through the kidneys. In contrast, an increase in the number of times you pass urine may be a warning of a possible infection. If you find yourself getting up during the night to go to the toilet, ask your doctor about it. Men may find that the problem is an enlarged prostate gland, which may also cause hesitancy in starting to urinate.

Cystitis, urethritis, and bladder infections make you want to empty the bladder frequently, but the amount of urine passed is often very small. Any swelling in the pelvis can press on the bladder and have the same effect. Frequency of urination is also an early sign of fibroids in the uterus and of pregnancy.

Involuntary urination

Accidental passing of urine when coughing, laughing, or sneezing is a common occurrence, especially in women. Called

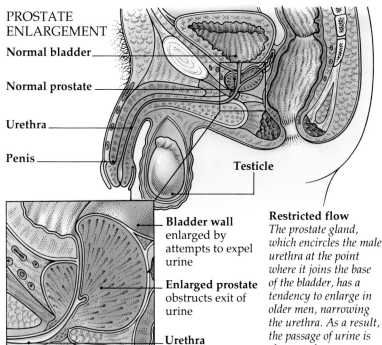

PROSTATE ENLARGEMENT
Normal bladder
Normal prostate
Urethra
Penis
Testicle

Bladder wall enlarged by attempts to expel urine

Enlarged prostate obstructs exit of urine

Urethra

Restricted flow
The prostate gland, which encircles the male urethra at the point where it joins the base of the bladder, has a tendency to enlarge in older men, narrowing the urethra. As a result, the passage of urine is obstructed.

stress incontinence, this is a condition that usually results from a weakening of the pelvic muscles, sphincters, and ligaments during pregnancy and childbirth. Incontinence may also occur because a person is unable to reach a toilet in time. Advancing age and some illnesses, such as a stroke, may cause temporary incontinence; a spinal injury can also affect bladder control in both the young and the old.

Beginning pelvic floor exercises immediately after childbirth helps to reduce incontinence and also prevents the problem from developing in the future. Learning to deliberately contract the sphincter muscles while urinating can improve bladder control. If incontinence persists, consult your doctor.

ABNORMAL URINE
If you have a bladder infection, your urine may become cloudy and dark, or it may take on a fishy smell. Some urinary problems, such as severe bladder infections, inflammation of the kidneys or bladder, or tumors in these organs, may cause you to pass blood, giving the urine a pink hue. This should always be reported to your doctor.

Avoiding embarrassment
The fear of an accident is one of the worst aspects of incontinence. One effective solution is to wear special underpants designed to carry a disposable, absorbent pad. This underwear is available for both men and women.

What is cystitis?

Cystitis is an inflammation of the inside of the bladder. It has a variety of symptoms, but sufferers do not necessarily experience them all at the same time.

You may feel a stinging or burning pain in the urethra when you pass urine. There may be a nagging urge to use the toilet, although once you reach it you may have very little urine to pass. Sometimes this urgency is accompanied by a frequency in the urge to urinate. Other symptoms include fever, an ache in the lower abdomen or back, tiredness, and cloudy urine. Blood in the urine may appear in severe cases.

What causes cystitis?

Your symptoms may be due to a variety of unrelated causes, including bacteria, an allergy to certain toiletries, friction or bruising of the urethra during sexual intercourse, a sensitive bladder, and even anxiety or depression. Common vaginal infections such as thrush can cause symptoms of cystitis, as can a parasitic infection and sexually transmitted diseases such as genital herpes.

Ureteral infection
If unchecked, the bacteria can enter the ureters and travel up to the kidneys.

Urethral infection
The bacteria multiply rapidly in the urethra, traveling up to the bladder.

Bladder infection
The bacteria irritate the lining of the bladder, causing inflammation.

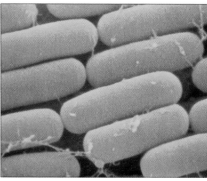

Bacteria of the bowel
The bacterium Escherichia coli, *photographed here by an electron microscope, is a common cause of cystitis.*

BACTERIAL CYSTITIS

Bacteria of the species *Escherichia coli,* which normally live harmlessly in the bowel, cause cystitis if they are spread to the urethra during sexual intercourse, by inserting tampons, by wiping yourself from back to front after a bowel movement, or even by wearing tight pants.

HOW TO PREVENT CYSTITIS

Whatever the cause of your cystitis, the following self-help measures will minimize the chance of recurrence:

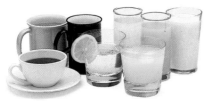

♦ Drink at least 3 or 4 pints of liquids every day. Women should drink cranberry juice to encourage acidity of the urine, which interferes with bacterial growth.

♦ Cystitis can be aggravated by coffee, tea, or alcohol. Try diluting them or avoid them altogether.

♦ Do not stop yourself from passing urine. After you urinate, count to 20 and then push out the remaining drops of urine.

♦ Always wipe yourself from front to back after going to the toilet to avoid spreading germs from the anus to the urethra.

♦ Wear cotton underwear to allow air to reach the genital area. Avoid wearing tight pants.

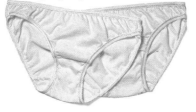

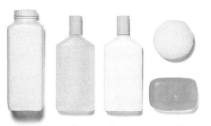

♦ Avoid using talcum powder, perfumed soaps, deodorants, or antiseptics in the genital area. Also, many bath oils, douches, bubble baths, and shampoos contain irritating chemicals.

♦ Urinating before and after sexual intercourse can prevent bacteria from being introduced into the urethra. A lubricant used during intercourse can prevent the bruising and swelling around the urethra that can lead to infection.

Candidiasis (thrush)
The fungus Candida albicans *(below) is responsible for the infection known as thrush. It causes a variety of symptoms, including white patches in the mouths of babies, rashes around the genitals of both women and men, and, most common, a thick, white vaginal discharge that is often accompanied by itching. The most effective treatment for vaginal candidiasis is an antifungal vaginal suppository or cream.*

GENITAL PROBLEMS

Infections and other disorders that affect the genitals occur more frequently in women than in men. The vagina is more susceptible to irritation by the chemicals used in toiletries and contraceptive products; incontinence may also provoke itching, caused by the urine.

Vaginal discharge

A clear discharge from the vagina is normal, but the amount and appearance of the discharge varies among women at different times during the menstrual cycle. If the discharge is excessive or has a strong odor, and if you feel soreness or itching, the vagina may be infected. First, make sure that you haven't forgotten to remove a tampon, which could be the cause of an extremely strong-smelling discharge. Otherwise, the discharge may be due to candidiasis (thrush), cystitis, trichomoniasis, or a sexually transmitted disease, such as gonorrhea or a chlamydial infection. Your doctor will take a vaginal (Pap) smear to identify the cause of the problem before prescribing the treatment you need. An infection may be cleared up with an antibiotic drug or antifungal drug. A reaction to a foreign body in the vagina, such as a forgotten tampon, clears up once the object has been removed.

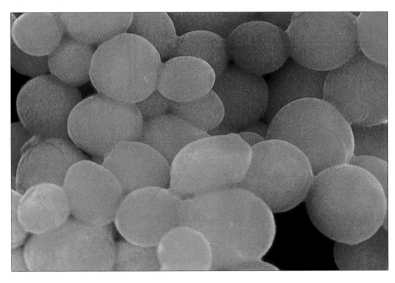

ASK YOUR DOCTOR URINARY AND GENITAL PROBLEMS

Q **One of my testicles seems to have enlarged over the past few weeks. Could this be cancer?**

A There are several causes of a swollen testicle, although cancer is a possibility. You may have a hydrocele, which is a fluid-filled sac surrounding the testicle. If the swelling is painful, you may have orchitis (inflammation of the testicle) or a twisted testicle. If the pain is severe, call your doctor now.

Q **The test results I've had for cystitis have been negative, but I still have a frequent urge to go to the toilet. What can I do now?**

A You may be suffering from what is known as urethral syndrome, in which the need to pass urine may be accompanied by discomfort in the lower abdomen and pain around the vulva. The most effective treatment is a high fluid intake combined with scrupulous personal hygiene. Herpes infections or internal problems such as pelvic inflammatory disease can also cause the symptoms you describe. If your symptoms persist despite a normal urine specimen, see your doctor.

Q **My partner has a discharge from his penis. Am I likely to catch anything from him?**

A Yes. This symptom may be due to gonorrhea or nonspecific urethritis, both of which are transmitted by sexual intercourse. Gonorrhea causes a discharge and vaginal soreness. Nonspecific urethritis may not produce any symptoms, but you could become a carrier. Both of you should see your doctor without delay.

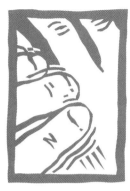

COMMON SKIN CONDITIONS

O NE PERSON IN FOUR consults a doctor about a skin disorder at some time in his or her life, but serious conditions are rare. Many skin disorders are simply cosmetic problems. Because changes in the skin are so easy to see, they can usually be recognized and treated at an early stage.

Disorders of the skin take on many shapes and can occur anywhere on the body. Even though skin cells are constantly being replaced as they wear out, the skin is extremely vulnerable. There are a huge number of skin disorders, but most of the common problems fall into several broad categories, including a variety of pimples, growths, rashes, and itchy conditions. Only the most common problems affecting the skin are discussed in this section.

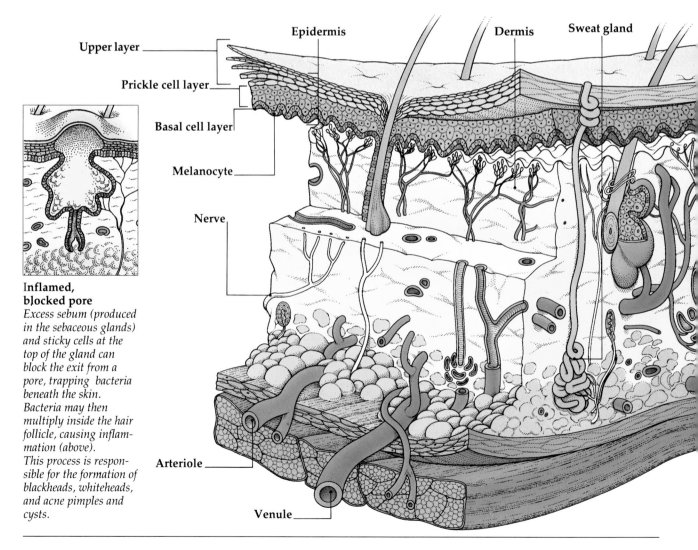

Inflamed, blocked pore
Excess sebum (produced in the sebaceous glands) and sticky cells at the top of the gland can block the exit from a pore, trapping bacteria beneath the skin. Bacteria may then multiply inside the hair follicle, causing inflammation (above). This process is responsible for the formation of blackheads, whiteheads, and acne pimples and cysts.

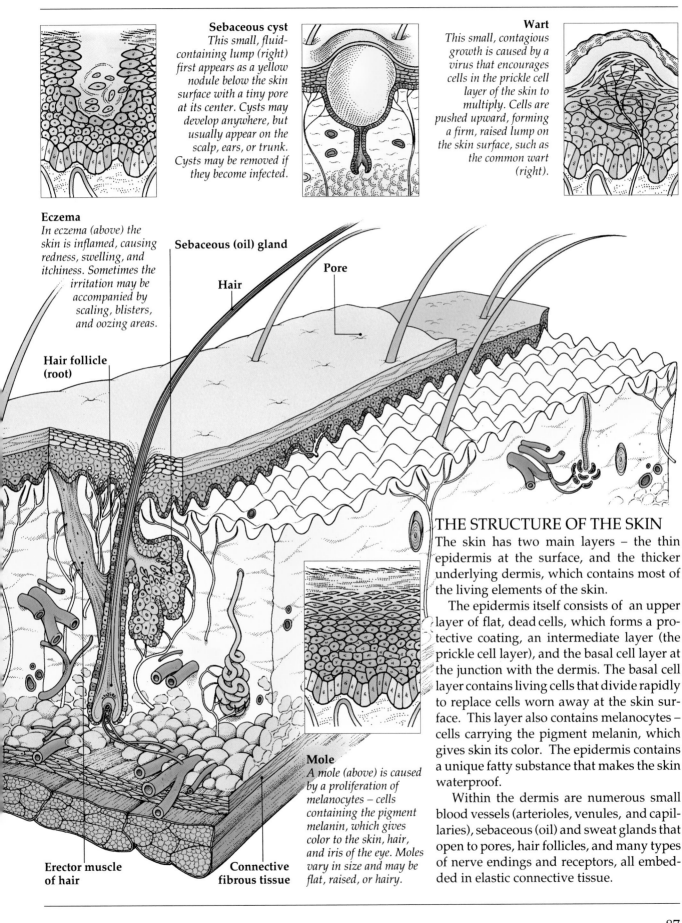

Sebaceous cyst
This small, fluid-containing lump (right) first appears as a yellow nodule below the skin surface with a tiny pore at its center. Cysts may develop anywhere, but usually appear on the scalp, ears, or trunk. Cysts may be removed if they become infected.

Wart
This small, contagious growth is caused by a virus that encourages cells in the prickle cell layer of the skin to multiply. Cells are pushed upward, forming a firm, raised lump on the skin surface, such as the common wart (right).

Eczema
In eczema (above) the skin is inflamed, causing redness, swelling, and itchiness. Sometimes the irritation may be accompanied by scaling, blisters, and oozing areas.

Sebaceous (oil) gland

Hair

Pore

Hair follicle (root)

Mole
A mole (above) is caused by a proliferation of melanocytes – cells containing the pigment melanin, which gives color to the skin, hair, and iris of the eye. Moles vary in size and may be flat, raised, or hairy.

Erector muscle of hair

Connective fibrous tissue

THE STRUCTURE OF THE SKIN

The skin has two main layers – the thin epidermis at the surface, and the thicker underlying dermis, which contains most of the living elements of the skin.

The epidermis itself consists of an upper layer of flat, dead cells, which forms a protective coating, an intermediate layer (the prickle cell layer), and the basal cell layer at the junction with the dermis. The basal cell layer contains living cells that divide rapidly to replace cells worn away at the skin surface. This layer also contains melanocytes – cells carrying the pigment melanin, which gives skin its color. The epidermis contains a unique fatty substance that makes the skin waterproof.

Within the dermis are numerous small blood vessels (arterioles, venules, and capillaries), sebaceous (oil) and sweat glands that open to pores, hair follicles, and many types of nerve endings and receptors, all embedded in elastic connective tissue.

MONITOR YOUR SYMPTOMS
BLEMISHES AND RASHES

There are many causes of skin eruptions. Among the most common are certain types of infectious illnesses, allergic reactions, and local skin irritation. These conditions may lead to the formation of groups of red or inflamed blemishes (flat or raised) and larger areas of inflamed skin. Although skin symptoms are not necessarily a sign of serious illness, it is wise to consult a doctor about the best treatment.

BEGIN HERE

Do you have one or more areas of red or spotted, but not blistered or tender, skin?

NO

YES

Infectious illnesses frequently produce rashes associated with fever.
Is your temperature raised?

NO

YES

SEE YOUR DOCTOR TODAY!

Call your doctor at once if a child has a rash and fever and is drowsy or confused.

Action Your doctor can usually make a precise diagnosis from the appearance and distribution of the rash and any additional symptoms. Other than acetaminophen (for children and teenagers under 16) or aspirin to reduce fever, no specific treatment is needed.

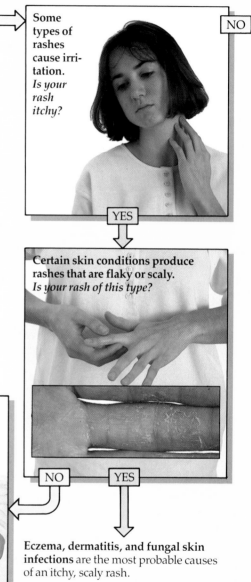

Some types of rashes cause irritation.
Is your rash itchy?

NO

YES

Certain skin conditions produce rashes that are flaky or scaly.
Is your rash of this type?

NO   YES

Rashes may be generalized areas of redness, or groups of individual spots.
Does your rash consist of several distinct, raised red spots?

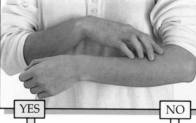

YES   NO

Insect bites may be the cause of your rash.

Action If calamine lotion does not provide adequate relief from itching, an over-the-counter antihistamine drug, taken by mouth, may be advised.

Eczema, dermatitis, and fungal skin infections are the most probable causes of an itchy, scaly rash.

Action Consult your doctor, who will determine the cause of your rash. Mild cases of eczema or dermatitis can often be relieved by a soothing emollient cream, while more severe cases may require treatment with a mild corticosteroid cream. Fungal infections are usually treated with an antifungal cream.

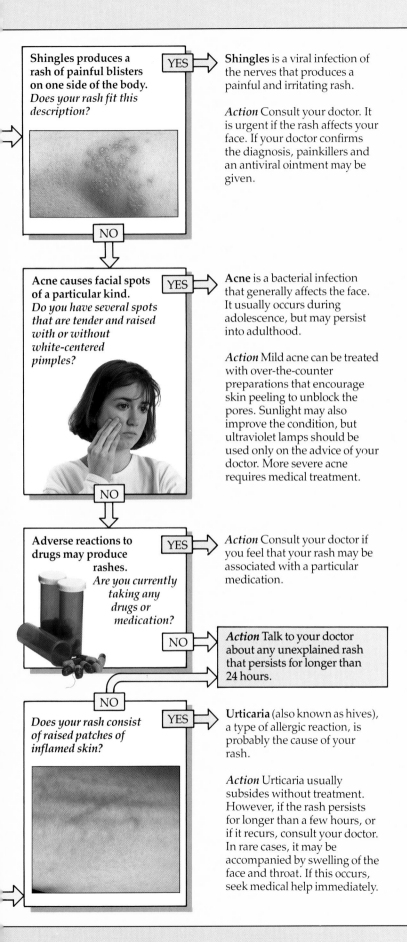

Shingles produces a rash of painful blisters on one side of the body. *Does your rash fit this description?* **YES** ⟹ **Shingles** is a viral infection of the nerves that produces a painful and irritating rash.

Action Consult your doctor. It is urgent if the rash affects your face. If your doctor confirms the diagnosis, painkillers and an antiviral ointment may be given.

NO

Acne causes facial spots of a particular kind. *Do you have several spots that are tender and raised with or without white-centered pimples?* **YES** ⟹ **Acne** is a bacterial infection that generally affects the face. It usually occurs during adolescence, but may persist into adulthood.

Action Mild acne can be treated with over-the-counter preparations that encourage skin peeling to unblock the pores. Sunlight may also improve the condition, but ultraviolet lamps should be used only on the advice of your doctor. More severe acne requires medical treatment.

NO

Adverse reactions to drugs may produce rashes. *Are you currently taking any drugs or medication?* **YES** ⟹ *Action* Consult your doctor if you feel that your rash may be associated with a particular medication.

NO ⟹ *Action* Talk to your doctor about any unexplained rash that persists for longer than 24 hours.

NO

Does your rash consist of raised patches of inflamed skin? **YES** ⟹ **Urticaria** (also known as hives), a type of allergic reaction, is probably the cause of your rash.

Action Urticaria usually subsides without treatment. However, if the rash persists for longer than a few hours, or if it recurs, consult your doctor. In rare cases, it may be accompanied by swelling of the face and throat. If this occurs, seek medical help immediately.

ACNE

Acne consists of small blackheads, whiteheads, red bumps, pustules, and cysts. It is caused by a combination of hormones, increased oily secretions and bacteria growth, and a stickiness of the pore openings. Pimples can form on the face, neck, shoulders, and back, causing extreme self-consciousness and, in severe cases, scarring.

There is no instant cure for acne. Because hormonal changes during puberty often increase the oiliness of the skin, acne is common in adolescents. The condition usually clears up by the middle 20s, but sometimes it persists. There is also a form of acne in women that occurs from the middle 20s until menopause. Diet has nothing to do with acne. Mild acne can be controlled by applying over-the-counter creams containing benzoyl peroxide or sulfur. Severe cases may respond to oral antibiotics or tretinoin, which reduce oil production in the sebaceous glands.

SKIN GROWTHS

There are many harmless skin growths, including warts, which are caused by a virus infection. Warts usually disappear in 2 to 4 years without treatment, but repeated applications of over-the-counter wart medicines can help remove them. Stubborn warts may need to be removed by a doctor, who may use liquid nitrogen, blistering medicines, acid, or a laser.

Other benign growths include papillomas (small, raised, flesh-colored growths), cutaneous horns (hard protrusions), and keratoses (scaly growths). Unlike warts, these skin growths are not contagious.

Most people have between 15 and 20 moles on their body. Occasionally, these pigmented growths become cancerous and must be removed. Most noncontagious growths require no treatment unless you wish to have them removed for cosmetic reasons.

How to recognize a malignant melanoma

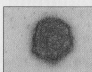

Mole

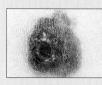

Malignant melanoma

A very small percentage of moles become cancerous (malignant melanomas). Check your moles with this "ABCD" test.

♦ **A for Asymmetry.** A common mole is nearly symmetrical.

♦ **B for Border.** A common mole has clear delineation of its color. If the color on one side of the mole blends into the surrounding skin, have the mole checked. Most moles are flat or evenly elevated. If one side of your mole becomes lumpy, have the mole checked.

♦ **C for Color.** Most moles are tan to dark brown and are evenly pigmented. Consult your doctor if a mole turns very dark brown, blue, or black, or if a dark mole suddenly has red, white, or blue in it.

♦ **D for Diameter.** Any mole larger than 6 mm should be checked.

ITCHING AND RASHES

Itching and rashes are not always caused by a skin disease. Sometimes, insect bites, allergies, or excessive dryness of the skin are responsible.

Inflammation of the skin is known as dermatitis. Many people suffer from a form of dermatitis, called eczema, that can cause severe itching. Eczema may be inherited, caused by an irritant, or due to an allergic reaction.

Itching may also be the result of infection by a virus or fungus. Chickenpox and scabies produce itchy rashes, and infections by the tinea group of fungi produce rings of red, scaly skin. The most common tinea infections are athlete's foot, which causes itching and cracking between the toes, and jock itch, in which a rash develops in the groin.

Relieving itching

If you have eczema, do not bathe in very hot water or use soaps or detergents. Emollient creams can help prevent your skin from drying out. Most forms of eczema respond to steroid creams, which your doctor may recommend.

HOW TO BEAT ATHLETE'S FOOT

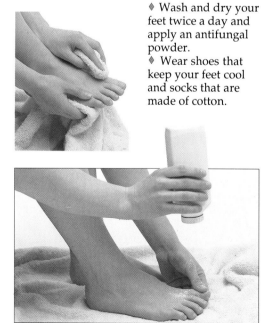

♦ Wash and dry your feet twice a day and apply an antifungal powder.

♦ Wear shoes that keep your feet cool and socks that are made of cotton.

ASK YOUR DOCTOR
COMMON SKIN COMPLAINTS

Q My sister-in-law told me that eczema has a tendency to run in families. Is this true?

A Eczema is so common that several cases may coincidentally occur in one family without the condition actually being inherited. In the case of infantile eczema, most affected babies have a family history of an allergic condition, such as eczema itself, asthma, or hay fever.

Q Is it true that eating chocolate and greasy foods like french fries causes acne?

A There is no medical evidence that any type of food can cause or aggravate acne.

Q I keep getting painful boils on the back of my neck. How can I stop them?

A Frequent skin infections are due to bacteria invading the skin. Keep your skin clean and don't pick at the boils. Some people are prone to ingrown hairs, which aggravate this condition. Oral antibiotics are often helpful.

Q My daughter has a red, oozing area of skin around her mouth and nose. It has a crust that looks like brown sugar. What can it be?

A It sounds as if your daughter has impetigo, a bacterial skin infection that is common in children. Impetigo is not harmful but is highly contagious, and may affect larger areas if left untreated. Consult your doctor, who may prescribe antibiotics or an ointment.

CASE HISTORY
A MYSTERIOUS RASH

AN ITCHY RASH **suddenly developed on the backs of both of Jim's hands. At first, small red patches appeared; within a few hours, the patches had spread over the whole hand and between his fingers. Several white spots also developed, and his hands began to look puffy. Worried that this might be a severe infection, Jim made an appointment to see his doctor.**

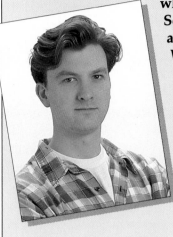

PERSONAL DETAILS
Name Jim McGowan
Age 26
Occupation Thermal window salesman
Family Father is well. Mother suffers from psoriasis.

MEDICAL BACKGROUND
Jim's records show that he had chickenpox as a child and mild acne during his teenage years. He has no history of serious skin disease.

THE CONSULTATION
Jim is worried that he has picked up a serious skin infection. He now has several fluid-filled blisters on his right hand, some of which have burst and released a clear fluid. Jim wants the skin to heal and be back to normal as soon as possible because he is concerned that his clients will be alarmed and repulsed by the appearance of his hands.

The doctor asks if Jim has been taking any medication, and whether he has had any skin problems in the past. He then questions Jim about his job and his hobbies, asking specifically about any substances his hands might have been in contact with in the last few days. The doctor then examines other areas of Jim's body, but finds that the rash is confined to the skin on his hands.

Jim tells the doctor that he had been working on an extension to his home over the past weekend when some cement splashed onto his hands. He thought nothing of it at the time and simply washed it off when he had finished.

THE DOCTOR'S IMPRESSION
Jim's rash is almost certainly ALLERGIC CONTACT DERMATITIS caused by contact with cement. Cement is a strong alkali that acts as an irritant on most people's skin. It may also be contaminated with chromate or cobalt, chemicals to which many people are sensitive. It is probable that Jim's skin became sensitized to the cement during a previous exposure, and that a severe rash will develop at the site of any future contact with this substance.

THE TREATMENT
The doctor prescribes a strong steroid cream, which Jim is instructed to apply to his hands three times a day. The doctor also writes a prescription for an antihistamine drug to take by mouth to relieve the itching and help Jim sleep at night. He is advised to wash his hands with a soap substitute, such as emulsifying ointment, while his skin is inflamed.

THE OUTCOME
After 2 weeks the skin looked less inflamed and the oozing areas had dried up. Jim was then prescribed a weaker steroid to reduce the risk of the side effects that can occur with prolonged use of a stronger preparation. After a month, he was able to return to work, although his skin remained dry and still had areas of scaling and crusting. Jim was warned that it could take several months for his skin to heal completely. In the meantime, he was advised to continue using a soap substitute and to wear heavy gloves if he worked with cement again.

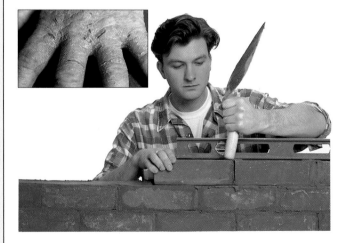

A severe rash
Jim had been building an extension to his home. When a painful red rash developed, he was unable to continue. Small red patches appeared on the backs of his hands and spread between his fingers. Eventually, painful cracks developed in several places.

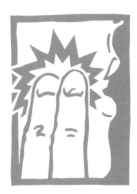

MOUTH AND TONGUE TROUBLES

ALL OF US OCCASIONALLY suffer from soreness or irritation of the mouth, lips, or tongue. In most cases, the cause is minor and the condition clears up within a few days. However, if you have a problem that persists for any length of time, or returns, it is wise to talk to your dentist or doctor about it.

Inspecting your mouth
Drinking alcohol and smoking increase the risk of mouth cancer. If you drink or smoke, it's a good idea periodically to examine the inside of your mouth in a mirror (below). Don't be afraid to show your doctor or dentist any persistent lump, ulcer, white patch, or change in the appearance of your tongue or gums.

Because many mouth and tongue problems represent a small part of more widespread disease, the condition of your mouth can be an important indicator of your health.

MOUTH ULCERS

A mouth ulcer is a break in the lining of the mouth that reveals the sensitive tissue underneath. Although they are not usually serious, mouth ulcers can be surprisingly painful for their size.

What causes mouth ulcers?
People often get single ulcers as a result of injuries from jagged teeth or ill-fitting dentures, or from eating

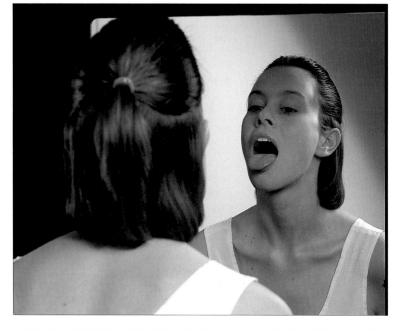

something hot. Small groups of ulcers, known as aphthous ulcers or canker sores, are also common. Some people find that they appear during times of stress or, in women, just before a menstrual period.

Most mouth ulcers heal by themselves within about 7 to 10 days. There is no treatment that is always effective. Rinsing your mouth with warm, salty water may help relieve pain; you can also buy anesthetic lozenges or ointment. Coating the ulcerated area with a special emollient before bedtime and after meals can help ease the pain and hasten healing. If you have particularly frequent recurrences, talk to your doctor.

MOUTH INFECTIONS

The lining of the mouth is highly resistant to infectious organisms. Most people do not get mouth infections unless they are run-down or eating nonnutritious foods. Occasionally, however, mouth ulcers are a sign of a more serious disease.

Cold sores
Many people are plagued by these recurrent crops of blisters on their lips and around their mouths.

Cold sores are a manifestation of herpes simplex, a viral infection that attacks almost everyone at some time in their lives. In a young child the original illness may pass unnoticed, but in older

WHERE DO PROBLEMS OCCUR IN THE MOUTH?

Various sores, ulcers, bumps, lumps, and areas of discoloration may affect any part of the mouth, lips, tongue, and gums. The chances of mouth problems developing can be minimized by practicing good oral hygiene, reducing the sugar content of your diet, avoiding smoking, reducing alcohol consumption, and having regular dental checkups.

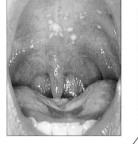

Thrush in roof of the mouth

Roof of the mouth
May be affected by thrush (white speckles) and by painful ulcers in the initial stages of a herpes attack.

Tongue
Inflammation and soreness may be caused by eating spicy food or may be a sign of anemia. The tongue may also be affected by canker sores, leukoplakia, and tumors.

Corners of the mouth
May be affected by thrush, causing painful cracking (angular cheilitis).

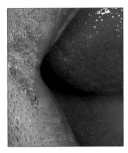

Angular cheilitis

Geographic tongue

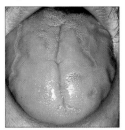

A persistent ulcer or lump on the tongue should always be checked by your doctor. Geographic tongue (red, shiny, flat patches and white patterns) and black hairy tongue (overgrowth and staining of the tongue) are two alarming but harmless conditions.

Gums
Gingivitis (inflammation of the gums) starts from bacterial plaque that adheres to the teeth and to the adjacent gum line. Unless treated, gingivitis may progress to cause destruction and ulceration of gum tissue, ultimately eroding the underlying bony sockets of the teeth.

Mouth lining
May be affected by thrush (raised, white speckles), ulcers caused by jagged teeth or dentures, canker sores, leukoplakia (white patches), oral lichen planus (a white, lacy network), and, in rare cases, a tumor.

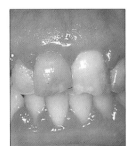

Gingivitis

Lips
The insides of the lips are a common site for aphthous ulcers, commonly called canker sores. They are small, round, yellow-gray, sore craters with an inflamed red border. Cold sores develop on or around the edges of the lips. They start as blisters, which break down to form painful, unsightly ulcers that crust over and take about 7 to 10 days to heal. The lip may also be a site for tumors.

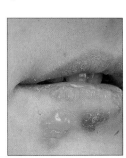

Cold sore

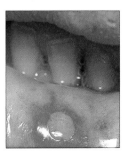

Canker sore

CANCER WATCH
Consult your doctor or dentist promptly if you discover any of the following changes in your mouth. Smokers and heavy drinkers should be especially alert for these conditions.

♦ Any persistent sore red patch
♦ Any white patch
♦ Any painless ulcer that spreads or won't heal
♦ Any new lump or swelling, whether or not it is growing, and whether or not it hurts.

people it causes fever, tender glands, and numerous tiny blisters. These blisters, which may appear on the gums and the roof of the mouth, eventually break down to form painful ulcers.

After the initial infection, the virus retreats up the nerves of the mouth, where it lies dormant within groups of nerve cells deep in the head. In some people, another infection (usually a cold), emotional stress, fatigue, strong sunlight, or even menstruation appears to reawaken the virus, which then travels down the nerve to the lip, causing the characteristic cold sores. The antiviral drug acyclovir can ease this condition but using the drug for long-term treatment to prevent a recurrence is not recommended. Sufferers should learn to recognize the burning feeling on the lip that heralds an attack; acyclovir relieves the symptoms best if it is applied as an ointment at an early stage.

Gum infections and thrush

Young adults who neglect their oral hygiene are at risk of necrotizing ulcerative gingivitis, a type of gum infection. This disease is more likely to occur if you are a smoker, are under stress, or have a throat or nose infection. The gums become sore, swollen, and bleed, and bacteria cause ulcers that break down the gum peaks between the teeth. Untreated areas are usually covered by a gray-white membrane that can be scraped off, leaving a raw, bleeding surface. Start treatment by careful cleansing with a soft toothbrush, but see your dentist promptly if you have any of the symptoms described here.

Many people harbor in their mouths the yeastlike fungus that causes thrush, usually without symptoms. If the fungus multiplies unchecked, it can be seen as creamy-white speckles, often on the inside of the cheeks and at the back of the mouth. Your whole mouth may also feel sore and dry. If you think you have thrush, see your doctor, who may be able to determine the probable cause and prescribe an effective antifungal medication.

HELPLINE
SORE MOUTH OR TONGUE

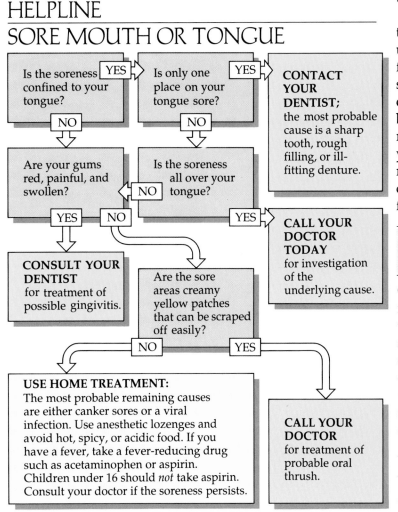

Is the soreness confined to your tongue? YES → **Is only one place on your tongue sore?** YES →

CONTACT YOUR DENTIST; the most probable cause is a sharp tooth, rough filling, or ill-fitting denture.

NO ↓ (gums) / NO ↓ (tongue)

Are your gums red, painful, and swollen?

Is the soreness all over your tongue? ← NO

YES →

CALL YOUR DOCTOR TODAY for investigation of the underlying cause.

YES / NO

CONSULT YOUR DENTIST for treatment of possible gingivitis.

Are the sore areas creamy yellow patches that can be scraped off easily?

NO / YES

USE HOME TREATMENT:
The most probable remaining causes are either canker sores or a viral infection. Use anesthetic lozenges and avoid hot, spicy, or acidic food. If you have a fever, take a fever-reducing drug such as acetaminophen or aspirin. Children under 16 should *not* take aspirin. Consult your doctor if the soreness persists.

CALL YOUR DOCTOR for treatment of probable oral thrush.

SORE TONGUE AND DRY MOUTH

General mouth soreness is uncommon in the absence of infection, but a sore tongue on its own is not uncommon. A sore tongue may be caused by a variety of mild forms of anemia, which can be confirmed by a blood test. An inflamed (red), smooth tongue is a more positive sign of anemia that should be promptly checked by your doctor.

What causes mouth dryness?

We all know that acute fear or anxiety dries up the mouth, so it's not surprising

HOW TO BEAT BAD BREATH (HALITOSIS)

Everyone wants to have pleasant-smelling breath. While bad breath is difficult to discern on your own, it often accompanies a bad taste in the mouth, which you can notice. Some of the primary causes of bad breath are listed here with suggestions for preventing and treating them. If bad breath persists, consult your doctor or dentist.

♦ **Foods such as garlic and onions.** Bad breath from eating these foods is caused by sulfur-based chemicals in the food that are absorbed into the bloodstream and exhaled through the lungs. The bad breath caused by these foods is not helped by mouth fresheners.

♦ **Smoking and alcohol consumption.** Using mouthwashes and thoroughly brushing the teeth may help lessen bad breath from these causes.

♦ **Bacteria** thriving on food particles between or around the teeth are a common and potent source of bad breath. Careful oral hygiene and regular teeth cleaning by a dentist or hygienist are needed. Brushing the tongue surface with a soft toothbrush will also help.

♦ **A dry mouth** may cause bad breath, which clears up after brushing your teeth or having a drink of water.

♦ **Prescribed drugs.** Some drugs cause bad breath; ask your doctor to tell you about them.

Cracks at the corners of the mouth
Sometimes thrush develops underneath a denture, especially if it is worn at night. The infected saliva causes painful cracks at the corners of the mouth. To avoid this, apply a nystatin ointment to the inside of your denture before inserting it.

that persistent anxiety can prolong mouth dryness. In addition, some prescription drugs reduce saliva production. If your prescription cannot be changed, a mouthwash may help.

Breathing through the mouth, especially at night, can dry out the front of your mouth and accelerate gum disease. Your dentist may prescribe a mouth guard to protect your gums. In general, the mouth becomes dryer with age, but some middle-aged to elderly people get a severe dry mouth and dry eyes, sometimes in conjunction with rheumatoid arthritis. This condition requires medical treatment.

ASK YOUR DOCTOR
MOUTH AND TONGUE TROUBLES

Q I'm pregnant and have heard that pregnancy could affect my gums. Is this true?

A When you're pregnant, and even at certain times during your menstrual cycle, hormonal changes can make your gums more prone to gingivitis. You may find that your gums are red and swollen and that they bleed easily when you brush your teeth. Be sure to have a checkup early in your second trimester.

Q My father has a white patch in his mouth that an oral surgeon wants to take a biopsy of. Does this mean he has mouth cancer?

A There are several possible causes of white patches in the mouths of older people, including heavy smoking and a type of chronic thrush infection. More rarely, a white patch can be due to a disorder called leukoplakia, a change in the mouth lining that may degenerate into cancer. This is why the specialist wants to remove a piece of the patch and have it examined.

Q My first baby was sick when she was teething. Can I prevent this in my next child?

A It's important to know that cutting teeth does not make a child sick. Your baby may get a little fussy and may drool more than usual, but he or she will not usually have any of the signs of a specific illness. Babies are a little more prone to infection around the time their primary teeth start to erupt. A child who is sick during teething should be seen by his or her pediatrician.

COMMON EYE AND VISUAL PROBLEMS

MOST EYE PROBLEMS are minor and do not carry any risk to your vision because they do not actually involve the optical structures; the common problems affect the external parts of the eye, such as the conjunctiva, lids, lashes, tear glands, and drainage ducts. However, the eye is a delicate organ that is easily damaged, so any concerns should be reported to an ophthalmologist.

Impaired vision most often becomes apparent when a person finds it difficult to read. More serious visual loss is usually the result of injury, infection, and, in older people, major disorders such as glaucoma, diabetic eye disease, or cataracts. If you have any of the symptoms listed in the WARNING box on page 98, call your ophthalmologist. However, most eye problems require less urgent testing or treatment.

Eyelid
The eyelids protect the eyes, but may be affected by cysts, styes, inturning, and outturning.

Tear glands
These glands produce tears that lubricate the eye.

Eye muscles

Conjunctiva
This transparent membrane, which covers the white of the eye and inner surfaces of the lids, may become irritated and inflamed.

Iris

Cornea
This transparent dome-shaped cap at the front of the eye, which is part of the eye's focusing equipment, is vulnerable to scratches or, more seriously, infection.

Tear ducts
The tear ducts drain tears from the eye. If they become blocked, the eye waters. The ducts can also become infected.

THE EYELIDS

The eyelids, which act as protective covers for the eye, are susceptible to a variety of problems.

Styes and cysts
Styes are tiny boils, or abscesses, that are caused by infection near the roots of the eyelashes. Once a stye  has started, you usually cannot halt its progress. When a yellow-white head has formed, recovery may be hastened by applying warm water compresses to help release the pus. Meibomian cysts are tight, pea-sized swellings in the eyelids. Each lid contains about 20 oil-producing glands with openings on the edge of the lid. If one of the glands becomes blocked, it is likely to form a cyst.

A meibomian cyst is harmless but may become infected and form an abscess. The cyst can be removed by an ophthalmologist.

Inturned eyelid

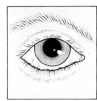

Known as entropion, an inturned eyelid is a common problem in older people. The edge of the eyelid turns inward, causing lashes to rub on the surface of the eyeball. This causes irritation and may result in conjunctivitis. Persistent entropion can cause permanent damage. Entropion is usually caused by aging changes of the structures of the eyelid. Gentle finger pressure can often restore the lid to its normal position but, if unsuccessful, it is sometimes necessary to have a minor operation to correct it.

Outturned eyelid

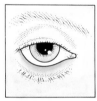

In this condition, called ectropion, the edge of the lid turns outward, away from the eyeball, and the exposed portion of the eyeball tends to become dry and sore. At the same time, there is excess watering of the eye because the tear ducts in the inner corners of the lower lids are out of position. Ectropion is usually caused by laxity of the edge of the lid and weakness of the muscle surrounding the eye. The condition may be treated by a minor operation to tighten the lid.

Trichiasis

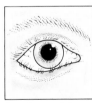

Trichiasis is a condition in which the lashes grow in an abnormal direction toward the eyeball. In this position, the lashes cause discomfort by rubbing on the surface of the eye. Pulling out the offending lashes is only a temporary solution to trichiasis. In fact, the resulting short, sprouting lashes may actually be more troublesome and painful than full-grown ones. If you have trichiasis , your doctor may recommend that you have minor surgery.

Blepharitis

Blepharitis is a persistent inflammation of the edges of the eyelid. If severe, it can cause abnormal growth or total loss of lashes. Blepharitis is often associated with dandruff, and lashes usually show greasy scales or crusts at skin level. If you think you have blepharitis, talk to your doctor, who may prescribe cleansing techniques or antibiotic and steroid ointments to treat this chronic condition.

THE FRONT OF THE EYE

The exposed surface of the white of the eye and the inner surface of the lids are lined by a sensitive, transparent membrane called the conjunctiva. The eyes are covered by a thin film of watery fluid called tears, which are produced by the lacrimal glands. In addition to being a sign of emotion, tears lubricate the eye and wash away any foreign bodies.

Eye irritation

Irritation is very common and may not be serious. It can be caused by excessive sunlight, a dusty atmosphere, cigarette smoke, allergy, mild infection, a foreign body under the upper lid, wearing your contact lenses for too long, or constantly rubbing your eyes. As long as your vision is not affected and you are not in pain, the problem can usually be solved by pinpointing and avoiding the cause. A minor blow to the eye can cause an alarming red area to appear in the conjunctiva. Talk to your doctor about this condition, which can sometimes be serious.

BLACK EYE

The skin surrounding the eye is loose, thin, and well supplied with veins that bleed easily if injured. Freed blood spreads readily under the skin and remains conspicuous until it is gradually removed by the natural process of absorption.

Contrary to popular mythology, raw steak has no effect on a black eye, which can take up to 3 weeks to heal, depending on the amount of blood released.

Using eye drops
Mild eye irritation can be soothed by the use of a variety of drops. Do not use eye drops too often, however, as they may aggravate the condition. Eye drops should be used only under the direction of your doctor.

Conjunctivitis

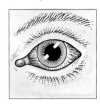

Conjunctivitis is an inflammation of the conjunctiva, the transparent membrane covering the eye. The eye becomes red and may water or produce a yellow discharge. Conjunctivitis has many causes, including infection, allergy (usually to pollen or cosmetics), heat, chemical irritation, radiation, and inability to close the eye. For conjunctivitis that is due to an irritant, avoid the cause. If there is any pain or disturbance of vision, or if the inflammation continues, see your doctor.

Dry eye

Dry eyes are due to a deficiency of tears. Feeling a sensation of dryness is very common. In many cases, however, the eyes are actually wet and the feeling may be due to irritation of the conjunctiva. Dry eyes require an ophthalmologist's examination because there is a danger of damage to the cornea and loss of sight. The use of artificial tear drops may be required for a short period or indefinitely.

Watery eye

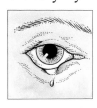

Continuous wetness of the eye may be the result of excessive tear production or of partial or total blockage of the tear drainage ducts. These ducts lead from the inner corners of the eyelids down into the back of the nose.

Excess tear production suggests an irritation or infection. However, tear duct blockage may occur in the newborn, in middle age, or later in life. It can be caused in infants by a delicate membrane obstructing a drainage duct. In adults, the duct may be blocked by an inflamed swelling or by the walls of the tear duct sticking together.

HELPLINE
RED EYE

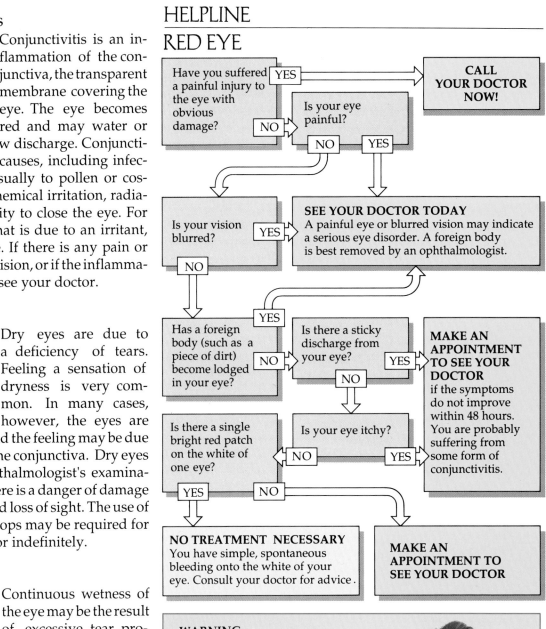

Have you suffered a painful injury to the eye with obvious damage? **YES** → **CALL YOUR DOCTOR NOW!**

NO → Is your eye painful? **YES** →

Is your vision blurred? **YES** →

SEE YOUR DOCTOR TODAY
A painful eye or blurred vision may indicate a serious eye disorder. A foreign body is best removed by an ophthalmologist.

NO →

Has a foreign body (such as a piece of dirt) become lodged in your eye? **YES** ↑

NO → Is there a sticky discharge from your eye? **YES** →

NO →

Is your eye itchy? **YES** →

MAKE AN APPOINTMENT TO SEE YOUR DOCTOR
if the symptoms do not improve within 48 hours. You are probably suffering from some form of conjunctivitis.

Is there a single bright red patch on the white of one eye? **NO** ←

YES →

NO →

NO TREATMENT NECESSARY
You have simple, spontaneous bleeding onto the white of your eye. Consult your doctor for advice.

MAKE AN APPOINTMENT TO SEE YOUR DOCTOR

WARNING

Consult your ophthalmologist if:
- There is a persistent change in the clarity of vision in either eye.
- You have a blind spot or loss of any part of your field of vision.
- You develop double vision.
- You see rainbow-colored rings around lights at night.
- You see spots, especially if they are reddish or brown.
- You see sparks, with or without eye movement.
- You have pain in your eye, especially if it is associated with blurred vision.
- Your eyes tear constantly.

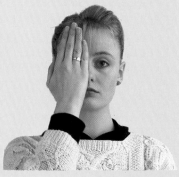

Checking your vision
By covering one eye at a time, you can determine whether or not an eye problem has affected your vision.

CASE HISTORY
A PAINFUL EYE

D R. FEINBERGER awoke one morning and found that his right eye was uncomfortable and watering. He had a constant feeling that there was something in his eye. This sensation was most noticeable when he blinked. He also realized that the white of his eye was getting increasingly red. At this stage, his vision wasn't affected, and he was too busy to take the time off to see his doctor. After 4 days, however, the vision in his right eye had become very blurred and he decided to call an ophthalmologist.

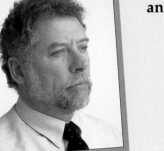

PERSONAL DETAILS
Name Karl Feinberger, PhD
Age 52
Occupation Engineer
Family No history of significant disease.

MEDICAL BACKGROUND
Dr. Feinberger has no medical history of any serious disorders and considers himself to be healthy. He is an expert marksman.

THE CONSULTATION
The ophthalmologist asks Dr. Feinberger to read a vision chart and finds that the vision in his right eye is seriously impaired.

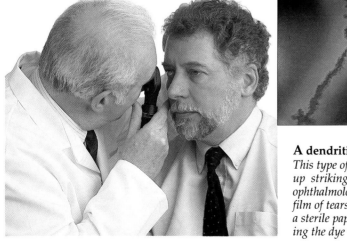

A microscopic examination of the eye shows a grayish, branching ulcer that resembles the veins of a leaf running across the center of the front of the right eye (cornea).

Through careful questioning, the doctor learns that, about 2 weeks before the onset of his symptoms, Dr. Feinberger had blown into his electric beard trimmer after using it and some dust had flown into his

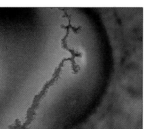

A dendritic ulcer
This type of ulcer shows up strikingly when the ophthalmologist touches the film of tears in the eye with a sterile paper strip containing the dye fluorescein.

right eye. The ophthalmologist also learns that Dr. Feinberger has recently had a cold sore on his lip.

THE OPHTHALMOLOGIST'S IMPRESSION
The appearance of the ulcer, known as a dendritic ulcer, strongly suggests to the ophthalmologist that it has been caused by the virus that causes herpes simplex, which is also present in cold sores.

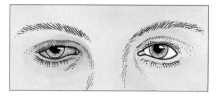

THE DIAGNOSIS
The ophthalmologist diagnoses a HERPES SIMPLEX VIRUS INFECTION. He takes material from the region of the ulcer to help confirm the diagnosis.

THE TREATMENT
After explaining what he is going to do, the ophthalmologist anesthetizes Dr. Feinberger's cornea with some painkilling drops and, using a sterile instrument, carefully rubs off a portion of the outer layer of the cornea, including the ulcer. He then puts some drops in the eye to prevent more inflammation, closes the eye, puts a pad over it, and prescribes an antiviral ointment. Dr. Feinberger will remove the pad and apply the ointment five times a day.

THE OUTCOME
The outer layer of the cornea, known as the epithelium, regenerates within a few days. The outlook depends on whether the virus has established itself in the deeper layers of the cornea. If, as in this case, it is still confined to the epithelium at the time of diagnosis, the ulcer usually heals, but may recur.

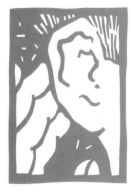

EAR AND HEARING DIFFICULTIES

SOME EAR PROBLEMS affect only the structural parts of the ear, while others affect hearing as well. Although ear problems can be distressing, most are not a serious cause for concern; your doctor can usually recommend a simple treatment.

The most common symptoms affecting the ears are earache and difficulty hearing. In addition, your sense of hearing can suffer interference from ringing, buzzing, and hissing sounds – a disorder known as tinnitus. In some cases, an ear problem can affect your sense of balance because the ear's semicircular canals, the organs in the inner ear that tell us whether we are balanced, can become infected by bacteria or a virus. This condition, known as labyrinthitis, causes feelings of nausea and vertigo (a spinning sensation).

EARACHE

Pain that is felt in the ear does not necessarily originate in the ear itself. Earache may be caused by a variety of conditions, including dental problems, tonsillitis, inflammation of the joint of the jaw, or neck injuries.

HOW WE HEAR SOUNDS

Sound travels through the air in waves. These waves are gathered by the pinna and funneled down the outer-ear canal to the eardrum. Sound waves striking the eardrum cause it to vibrate. The vibrations then pass through the middle-ear cavity to the inner ear via three tiny interconnecting bones – the hammer, anvil, and stirrup. Once inside the inner ear, the vibrations reach the cochlea, an organ that transforms them into nerve impulses and sends them through to the brain via the auditory nerve. The brain then identifies the sounds by referring them to a "memory bank" of past experiences of that sound.

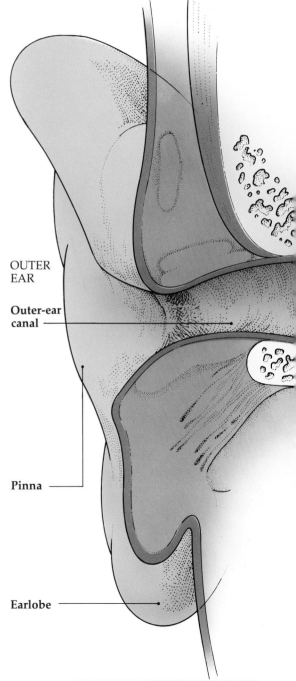

OUTER EAR

Outer-ear canal

Pinna

Earlobe

Outer ear
The outer ear consists of the pinna and the ear canal, which funnel sound waves toward the eardrum. The canal can become infected, producing pain and a discharge. Hearing difficulties can occur if the canal becomes blocked with excess earwax.

WHERE DO EAR PROBLEMS OCCUR?

The ear consists of three main sections: the outer ear, middle ear, and inner ear. Generally, disorders of the outer ear are not serious, although a boil or abscess in the outer-ear canal can be extremely painful. The middle ear is prone to both viral and bacterial infection, especially if you are suffering from a cold. Disorders of the very delicate organs of the inner ear – the cochlea and labyrinth – may be much more serious, sometimes resulting in complete loss of hearing.

Labyrinth
The labyrinth is a group of fluid-filled canals that controls balance. Disorders of the labyrinth include viral infection (labyrinthitis) and Meniere's disease, an increase in the amount of fluid in the canals. Both produce dizziness and nausea.

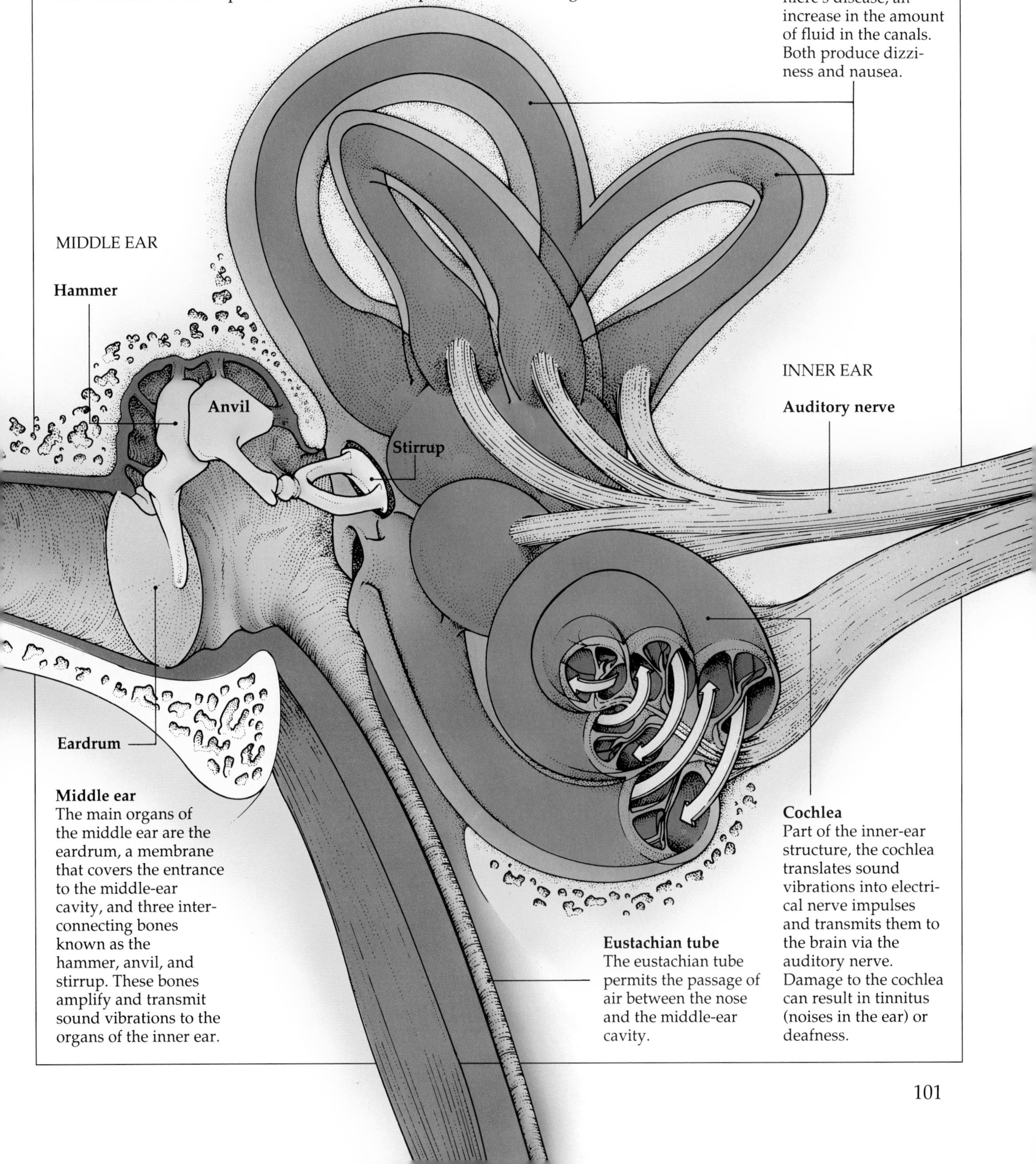

MIDDLE EAR

Hammer

Anvil

Stirrup

INNER EAR

Auditory nerve

Eardrum

Middle ear
The main organs of the middle ear are the eardrum, a membrane that covers the entrance to the middle-ear cavity, and three interconnecting bones known as the hammer, anvil, and stirrup. These bones amplify and transmit sound vibrations to the organs of the inner ear.

Eustachian tube
The eustachian tube permits the passage of air between the nose and the middle-ear cavity.

Cochlea
Part of the inner-ear structure, the cochlea translates sound vibrations into electrical nerve impulses and transmits them to the brain via the auditory nerve. Damage to the cochlea can result in tinnitus (noises in the ear) or deafness.

101

MONITOR YOUR SYMPTOMS
PAIN IN THE EAR

Earache is a symptom that occurs more often in children than in adults. Whether the pain is dull and throbbing or sharp and stabbing, all severe or persistent earaches require medical attention.

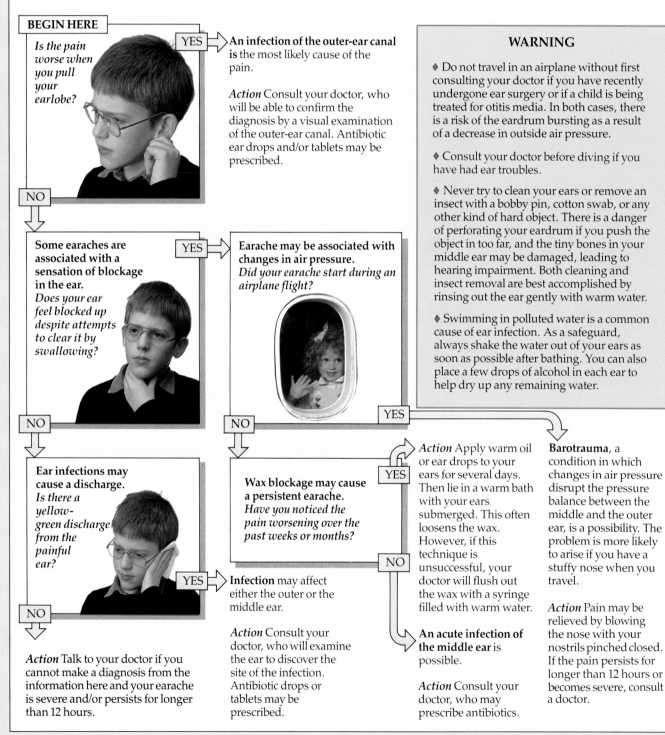

BEGIN HERE

Is the pain worse when you pull your earlobe? **YES** ➡

An infection of the outer-ear canal is the most likely cause of the pain.

Action Consult your doctor, who will be able to confirm the diagnosis by a visual examination of the outer-ear canal. Antibiotic ear drops and/or tablets may be prescribed.

NO ⬇

Some earaches are associated with a sensation of blockage in the ear. *Does your ear feel blocked up despite attempts to clear it by swallowing?* **YES** ➡

Earache may be associated with changes in air pressure. *Did your earache start during an airplane flight?*

NO ⬇ / **YES**

NO ⬇

Ear infections may cause a discharge. *Is there a yellow-green discharge from the painful ear?* **YES** ➡

Infection may affect either the outer or the middle ear.

Action Consult your doctor, who will examine the ear to discover the site of the infection. Antibiotic drops or tablets may be prescribed.

NO ⬇

Action Talk to your doctor if you cannot make a diagnosis from the information here and your earache is severe and/or persists for longer than 12 hours.

Wax blockage may cause a persistent earache. *Have you noticed the pain worsening over the past weeks or months?* **YES**

Action Apply warm oil or ear drops to your ears for several days. Then lie in a warm bath with your ears submerged. This often loosens the wax. However, if this technique is unsuccessful, your doctor will flush out the wax with a syringe filled with warm water.

NO

An acute infection of the middle ear is possible.

Action Consult your doctor, who may prescribe antibiotics.

Barotrauma, a condition in which changes in air pressure disrupt the pressure balance between the middle and the outer ear, is a possibility. The problem is more likely to arise if you have a stuffy nose when you travel.

Action Pain may be relieved by blowing the nose with your nostrils pinched closed. If the pain persists for longer than 12 hours or becomes severe, consult a doctor.

WARNING

♦ Do not travel in an airplane without first consulting your doctor if you have recently undergone ear surgery or if a child is being treated for otitis media. In both cases, there is a risk of the eardrum bursting as a result of a decrease in outside air pressure.

♦ Consult your doctor before diving if you have had ear troubles.

♦ Never try to clean your ears or remove an insect with a bobby pin, cotton swab, or any other kind of hard object. There is a danger of perforating your eardrum if you push the object in too far, and the tiny bones in your middle ear may be damaged, leading to hearing impairment. Both cleaning and insect removal are best accomplished by rinsing out the ear gently with warm water.

♦ Swimming in polluted water is a common cause of ear infection. As a safeguard, always shake the water out of your ears as soon as possible after bathing. You can also place a few drops of alcohol in each ear to help dry up any remaining water.

These disorders sometimes cause earache by transmitting pain signals along the nerves in the head that end in the same region of the brain as those coming from the ear. It is this kind of "referred" earache that children often suffer when they are teething. Adolescents may also feel pain in the ear when their wisdom teeth are erupting.

The most common cause of earache, however, is an infection, which can occur in the outer and middle parts of the ear. In an outer-ear infection, the skin lining the tube that leads to the eardrum becomes infected – a condition called otitis externa. This disorder becomes particularly painful if a small boil develops at the site of infection.

Pain in the middle ear

The middle ear is sealed from the outer-ear passage by the eardrum. If the air pressure inside and outside the eardrum is unequal, the eardrum is stretched and an earache can develop.

Descending in an airplane, or even in an elevator, can sometimes cause pain in the ears because the changing pressure outside the eardrum is not matched within. Called barotrauma, the condition can be remedied by chewing gum or by blowing the nose with the nostrils pinched. A similar pain may be caused by middle-ear infection leading to otitis media (see below). In this case, inflammation and swelling of tissues in the ear raise the pressure in the middle ear.

HEARING DIFFICULTIES

Problems with hearing can stem from a number of sources. The cause of hearing loss is usually a temporary blockage of the outer or middle ear, and hearing is restored when the blockage is removed. Certain drugs, however, may cause hearing loss when taken in large doses. Known as ototoxic drugs, they include the aminoglycoside antibiotics streptomycin, gentamicin, and tobramycin. In-

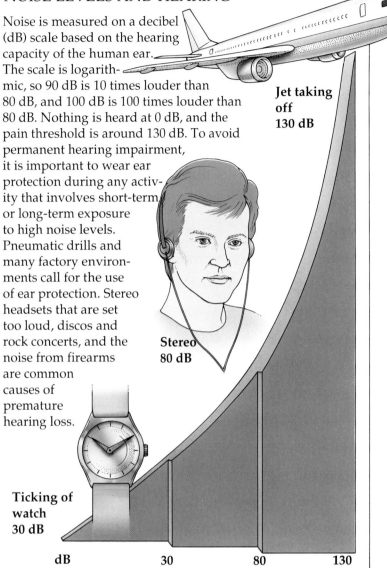

NOISE LEVELS AND HEARING

Noise is measured on a decibel (dB) scale based on the hearing capacity of the human ear. The scale is logarithmic, so 90 dB is 10 times louder than 80 dB, and 100 dB is 100 times louder than 80 dB. Nothing is heard at 0 dB, and the pain threshold is around 130 dB. To avoid permanent hearing impairment, it is important to wear ear protection during any activity that involves short-term or long-term exposure to high noise levels. Pneumatic drills and many factory environments call for the use of ear protection. Stereo headsets that are set too loud, discos and rock concerts, and the noise from firearms are common causes of premature hearing loss.

Jet taking off 130 dB

Stereo 80 dB

Ticking of watch 30 dB

dB   30   80   130

flammation of the middle ear, known as otitis media, also causes hearing loss and is very common. Inflammation occurs when bacteria from a respiratory infection, such as a cold, travel up the eustachian tube from the throat and inflame the tissues of the middle ear. If the tube then becomes blocked, fluids and pus produced by the infection cannot drain. The fluids accumulate, causing hearing loss by inhibiting the vibration of the eardrum.

Children are particularly prone to otitis media because their eustachian tubes are short and infection can easily reach the middle ear. Otitis media may

ASK YOUR DOCTOR
EAR AND HEARING
DIFFICULTIES

Q I have had a discharge from my ear for some weeks, but can still hear quite well. Should I worry?

A The discharge could be coming from an infection of the outer-ear canal or from a middle-ear infection in which pressure has perforated the eardrum. If your eardrum is perforated, you may not notice any hearing loss, but it is still advisable to see your doctor for treatment.

Q My aunt suffers from Meniere's disease. What is it, and is there anything she can do about it?

A Meniere's disease is a condition in which there is an increase of pressure in the fluid of the inner ear. This increase in pressure damages both the hearing and balancing mechanisms, so your aunt may suffer sudden dizziness and spatial disorientation. Other symptoms are nausea, vomiting, hearing loss, and tinnitus in the affected ear. Your aunt may feel normal between attacks, which tend to become more frequent and more severe. Meniere's disease is treated with a variety of drugs. If drugs are not successful, surgery may be needed to relieve the pressure.

Q My little boy has a deformed ear. Will it affect his ability to hear normally?

A The inner ear and the outer ear develop separately, so there is a good chance that his hearing is normal. Nevertheless, you should take him to an ear, nose, and throat specialist for testing. Cosmetic surgery can be used to repair his ear and help his self-esteem.

Earwax
A secretion from the ceruminous glands in the outer ear may accumulate and harden to form earwax, which can plug the ear and prevent sound waves from reaching the eardrum. Earwax blockage is a common cause of temporary hearing loss, particularly in the elderly.

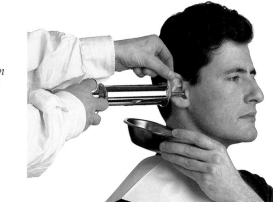

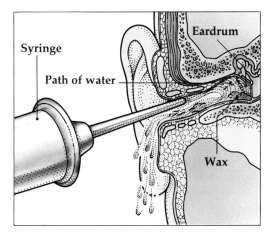

Syringe

Path of water

Eardrum

Wax

Removing earwax
Earwax is removed in the doctor's office by syringing. To avoid pushing the wax against your eardrum, the doctor uses the syringe to direct a stream of a warm solution into the roof of each ear canal. As the liquid washes out, it brings the wax with it. The liquid drains into a dish that is held next to your ear.

cause mild discomfort with few symptoms or it can become an acute illness with high fever and severe pain. Antibiotics are used to treat middle-ear infections. If left unattended, the pressure of the fluids can burst the eardrum.

Noises in the ears

Constant sounds in the ear, such as ringing, hissing, buzzing, or a noise like waves crashing, are called tinnitus. These sounds are the result of damage to the cochlea, the most sensitive component of the hearing mechanism. Reactions to tinnitus vary from person to person – some people are able to ignore the disability, while others are driven into deep depression by it. Tinnitus is sometimes treated by the installation of a special hearing aid designed to mask the annoying sounds. The hearing aid helps about 15 percent of the people who use it. Simpler remedies include playing a radio in the background to try to mask the tinnitus.

HEARING LOSS AND OLD AGE

As people get older, their hearing may lose sensitivity, especially to high tones, which can cause difficulty in understanding speech, even if it is loud. A high-tone hearing loss also interferes with understanding speech when there is noise in the background. Hearing that is impaired in this way can often be helped by a hearing aid that enhances the high tones. Do not assume, however, that your hearing loss is due to age without a full assessment by an ear specialist.

CASE HISTORY
HEARING LOSS

WELL-LIKED BUT **regarded as "the slow one" by her family, Carol spent several years struggling to overcome a hearing impediment without anyone, including herself, being aware that she had one. One day, while treating her younger sister in his office, the family doctor asked Carol how her science project was coming along. He realized that Carol apparently could not hear what he was saying.**

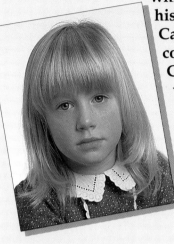

PERSONAL DETAILS
Name Carol Komski
Age 7
Occupation Student
Family No history of significant disease.

MEDICAL BACKGROUND
Carol has suffered many colds and bouts of tonsillitis, for which she has been prescribed numerous courses of antibiotics. She is underweight and small for her age. At school she is described as inattentive and her performance is well below average.

THE CONSULTATION
The doctor speaks to Carol again, this time more loudly, and asks her whether she ever has earaches. Carol says "no." The doctor checks her eardrums with a flashlight and finds them both to be yellow, rather than clear, with some dilated blood vessels. They are immobile, which makes them unresponsive to sound.

Examining her further, the doctor finds that her adenoids (tissues lying at the back of the nose) are so large that she is almost unable to breathe through her nose. The openings to her eustachian tubes are blocked. When the doctor holds a vibrating tuning fork close to her ear, she hears it only faintly, but she shows delight when the base of the tuning fork is pressed against the mastoid bones that lie behind each ear.

FURTHER INVESTIGATION
The doctor gives Carol a pure-tone audiogram test. Her results indicate a degree of hearing loss that would render speech muffled and would make it very difficult to hear.

THE DIAGNOSIS
Carol is suffering from SECRETORY OTITIS MEDIA. Both of her middle ears contain a sticky, gluey substance that is preventing movement of the eardrums and the chain of three tiny bones inside her middle ear. Carol's enlarged adenoids had prevented the material from draining out through the eustachian tubes into the back of her throat.

THE TREATMENT
A week later, Carol has her adenoids removed. The material in her middle ears is sucked out through a small incision in each eardrum, and a small tube is placed in each cut to maintain drainage. No infection is found in her middle ears.

THE OUTLOOK
Carol's hearing is fully restored, and it soon becomes apparent that the hearing loss from the middle-ear problem had caused her slow progress at school. She is also able to breathe freely through her nose.

Tuning-fork test
Tuning forks are used to determine whether a patient is suffering from conductive deafness, in which sounds are unable to reach the inner ear due to a mechanical defect in the middle ear, or sensorineural deafness, in which hearing loss is caused by nerve impulses not being passed on to the brain from the inner ear.

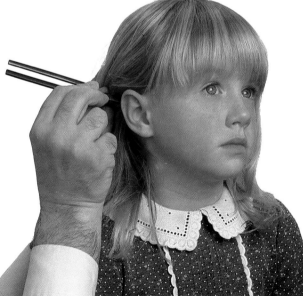

CHAPTER THREE

TAKING CARE OF YOUR BODY

INTRODUCTION

STAYING TRIM

MAINTAINING
YOUR SKIN
AND HAIR

CARING
FOR YOUR
TEETH AND EYES

A FINELY TUNED and well-maintained body is important for two reasons: it promotes a feeling of well-being and health and it looks good. All the visible parts of your body – your skin, hair, eyes, hands, and teeth – as well as your overall body shape, are effective reflectors of how healthy you are. But they don't, for the most part, take care of themselves. They require some attention from you. It's easy to dismiss body maintenance as being the province of those with plenty of time and money at their disposal. But it needn't be. Taking care of yourself is neither frivolous nor a waste of your time. There are enormous benefits to be gained in terms of your morale and happiness, with corresponding benefits for your health and your quality of life. Of course, no one is entirely happy with his or her physical makeup. There are many things over

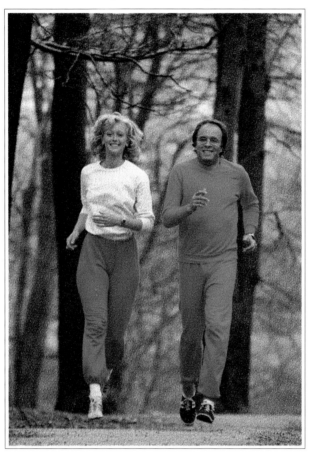

which we have no control, such as our height, the size of our feet, the shape of our bones, and the color of our eyes. What is important is to make the best of what we have and to capitalize on our good points. One vital statistic over which we do have some control is our weight, yet studies have shown that about one quarter of adult men and one third of adult women in the US are overweight – that is, more than 20 percent over the ideal weight for their height. Our section in this chapter on staying trim emphasizes the importance of proceeding slowly when trying to lose weight, while maintaining a balance of nutritious foods. Reducing the intake of fat in your diet is important; it can be achieved through some simple alterations in the way you select and cook your food. Caring for your skin, hair, eyes, and teeth can also pay dividends over both the short and long term. Avoiding too much sun exposure, for example, not only prevents the immediate effects of painful sunburn and peeling skin – but may also prevent a skin cancer from developing later on. Regular attention to your teeth keeps your breath fresh today and can save you expensive and possibly painful dental treatment, or need for dentures, tomorrow. If you wear contact lenses, a few extra minutes devoted to the care and cleaning of your lenses each day can make the difference between healthy eyes and infected ones. Taking care of yourself doesn't have to take hours of your time. Just a few minutes every day can make all the difference in the way you look and feel. The important idea is to accept that you are worth it. Don't neglect your body until it becomes a problem. The benefits will last a lifetime.

STAYING TRIM

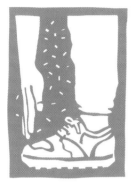

ALL OF US SHOULD KNOW the body weight that is best suited to our life-style and physique. Maintaining your weight can be difficult. However, when you do, your body is healthier and more efficient. And the rewards of weight control will be evident in the way you feel and present yourself.

Checking your weight
To determine whether you are in the underweight range, the normal weight range, or the overweight range (more than 20 percent over your desirable weight), first find your height on the left side of the chart below. Then run your finger across to your current weight. The shaded areas on the figures below indicate where fat can accumulate.

In today's sedentary society, we are often encouraged to indulge ourselves in more of everything than we really need. When it comes to food, the consequence of overindulgence and labor-saving life-styles is an increase in body weight. Over a period of time, being overweight can place serious strain on the heart, bone structure, and digestive system. Conversely, desperate attempts to avoid obesity may lead us to eat poorly and much less than the body needs, resulting in fatigue, malnutrition, and a slow wasting away of the body.

WEIGHT AND HEALTH

To confirm whether your current weight is appropriate for your height, refer to the height/weight charts on this page. Ideally, your weight should remain more or less the same after the age of 25. However, most people gain a little as they grow older, reaching their maximum weight at around the age of 50.

About 20 to 25 percent of the weight of an average adult woman is fat; fat accounts for between 10 and 20 percent of

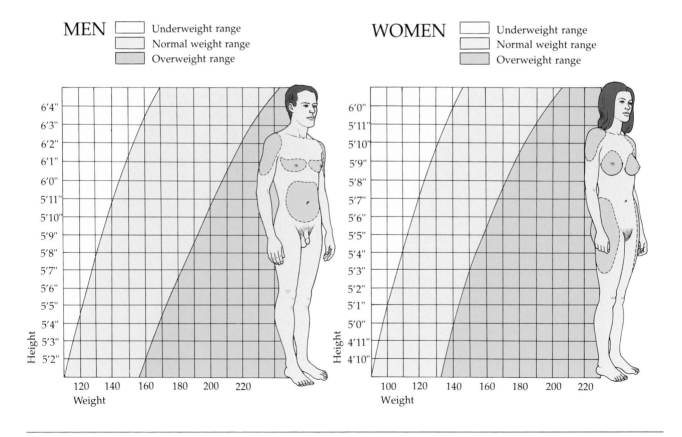

MEN
☐ Underweight range
▨ Normal weight range
▨ Overweight range

WOMEN
☐ Underweight range
▨ Normal weight range
▨ Overweight range

the weight of the average adult man. Any more fat than this is both unnecessary and unhealthy.

People who are overweight are more vulnerable than trim people to coronary heart disease, diabetes, stroke, hernias, gallbladder trouble, and cancer, notably cancer of the colon and rectum. Overweight people also tend to have less energy than those of ideal weight.

Life expectancy
Seriously underweight and overweight people die earlier than their trimmer counterparts. Statistics suggest that a person who is more than 40 percent over his or her desirable weight runs twice the risk of dying of coronary heart disease. Someone who is 20 to 30 percent over his or her desirable body weight may be three times more likely to die of diabetes than a person whose body weight falls within a desirable range.

MAINTAINING YOUR WEIGHT

Keeping your weight at the correct level involves adequate exercise and careful attention to diet. It is easy to gain several pounds without even realizing it. Most people need to adjust their diet occasionally and exercise more to compensate.

How should I diet?
The golden rule in dieting is to proceed slowly, never attempting to lose more than 2 pounds in a week. If you exceed that target, your weight loss will be in fluids and muscle, rather than in fat.

It is not advisable to limit yourself to a diet of only a few foods; a highly restricted diet requires that you pay more attention to the composition of your daily meals. Ideally, you should choose from the widest possible variety of fresh fruits and vegetables, lean meats and fish, and whole-grain products. Eat high-fiber, low-fat foods and avoid pastries and sweets as much as possible.

HOW TO AVOID OVEREATING
◆ Choose a smaller plate than usual and eat slowly.
◆ Avoid large meals just before bedtime.
◆ Weigh yourself regularly; if your weight increases, cut down on your food intake and exercise more.
◆ Eat three small meals a day rather than two large ones. If you are still hungry, you can fill up on whole-grain bread and fluids, such as water and fruit juices. A day's diet of delicious, low-fat, low-calorie foods is shown below.

Breakfast
Citrus fruit; unsweetened cereal with low-fat milk; and whole-grain bread with a pat of low-fat spread and preserves.

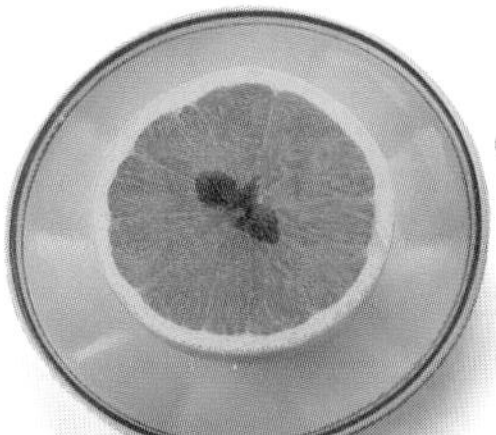

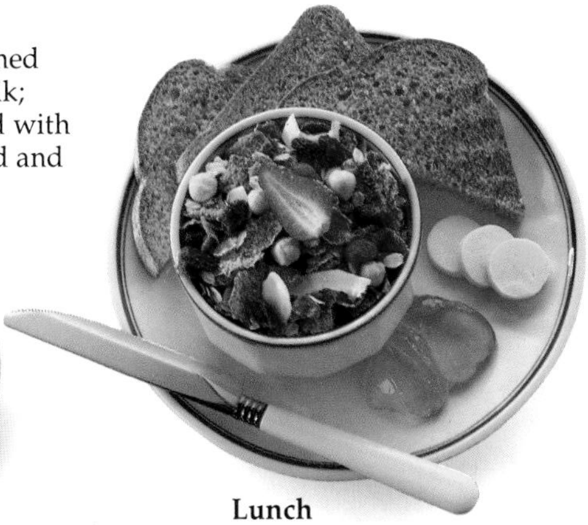

Lunch
Soup; salad of mixed greens and fresh vegetables with a low-calorie dressing; sandwich with lean meat, onion, lettuce, and tomato.

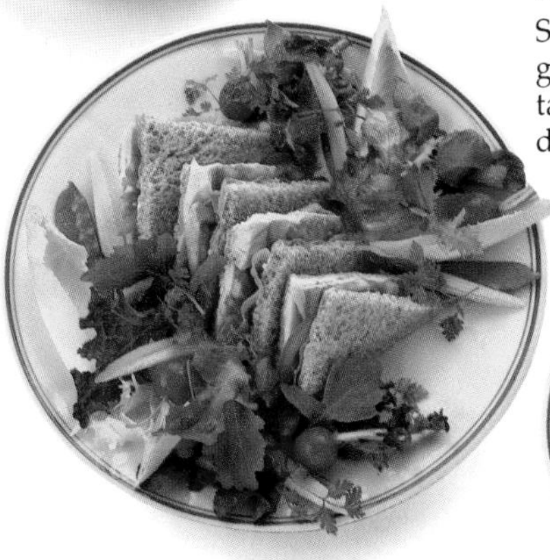

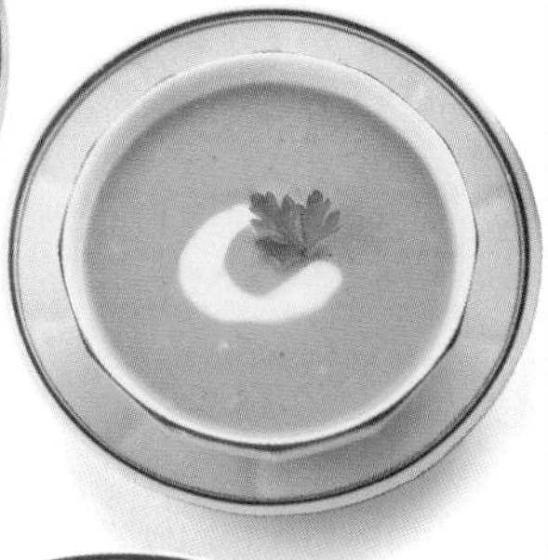

Dinner 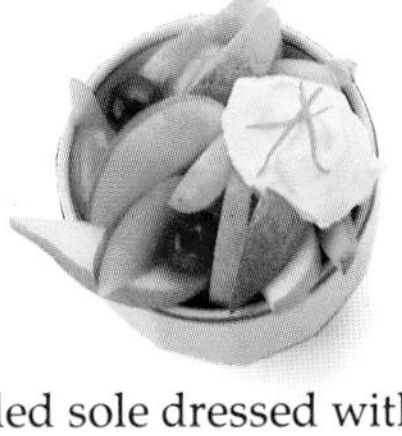 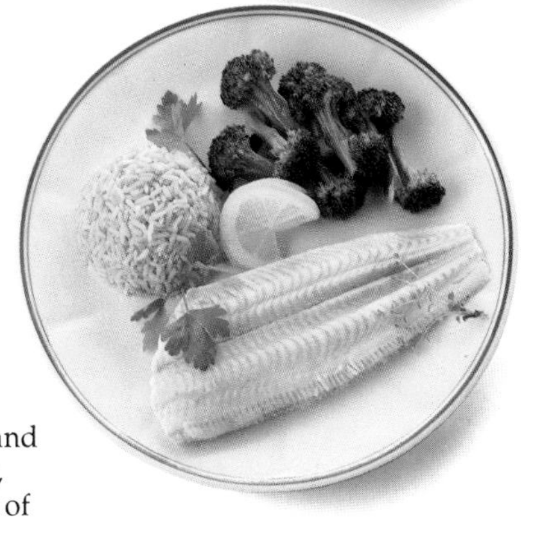
Broiled sole dressed with thyme, parsley, and lemon juice served with steamed broccoli and rice with soy sauce; fruit salad of apples, pears, peaches, and grapes served with yogurt, cottage cheese, or a wedge of cheese.

REDUCING YOUR FAT INTAKE

When you diet to lose weight, it is neither desirable nor necessary to eliminate altogether foods that contain fats. As shown in the table below, if you choose low-fat versions of each food, or prepare the foods in a certain way, you can still enjoy your favorite meals without incurring the penalty of a high fat intake. Remember: fat is energy-dense – 9 kilocalories (kcal) per gram.

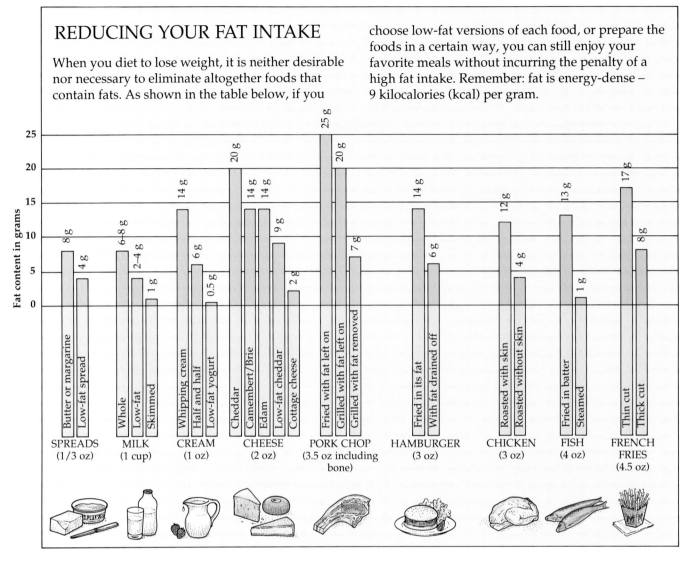

Fat content in grams

SPREADS (1/3 oz)	Butter or margarine — 8 g	Low-fat spread — 4 g	
MILK (1 cup)	Whole — 6–8 g	Low-fat — 2–4 g	Skimmed — 1 g
CREAM (1 oz)	Whipping cream — 14 g	Half and half — 6 g	Low-fat yogurt — 0.5 g
CHEESE (2 oz)	Cheddar — 20 g	Camembert/Brie — 14 g	Edam — 14 g
	Low-fat cheddar — 9 g	Cottage cheese — 2 g	
PORK CHOP (3.5 oz including bone)	Fried with fat left on — 25 g	Grilled with fat left on — 20 g	Grilled with fat removed — 7 g
HAMBURGER (3 oz)	Fried in its fat — 14 g	With fat drained off — 6 g	
CHICKEN (3 oz)	Roasted with skin — 12 g	Roasted without skin — 4 g	
FISH (4 oz)	Fried in batter — 13 g	Steamed — 1 g	
FRENCH FRIES (4.5 oz)	Thin cut — 17 g	Thick cut — 8 g	

How many calories do I need?

Many people are fat because their food intake far exceeds their energy requirements. But, just as important, they often eat inappropriate foods, particularly those that are rich in calories but add little to the nutritional value of their meals. These calories are known as "empty" calories.

Most active people lose weight on an intake of about 1,200 to 1,500 calories a day. Cutting out excess fat is often all that is necessary. Starvation diets that are designed to drastically reduce your food intake should be avoided. They are disruptive to your digestive system and are seldom successful in achieving long-term weight loss because they create a craving for food that often results in binges and rapid weight gain. Also, for most people, a diet of less than 1,200 calories a day involves an increased risk of nutritional deficiencies.

Why should I exercise?

Exercising allows you to eat a more varied diet and speeds up the rate at which pounds are shed. It ensures that fat, and not muscle, is reduced. Exercise also helps weight loss by directing your attention away from the large amounts of high-calorie snack foods that so often accompany inactivity.

The type of exercises you choose depends largely on your age and health, but it is important to pick those that you

WARNING
Very low calorie diets (liquid formula diets of less than 500 calories a day) are available for extremely obese people who have not been able to lose weight on diets. These diets should be used only under medical supervision.

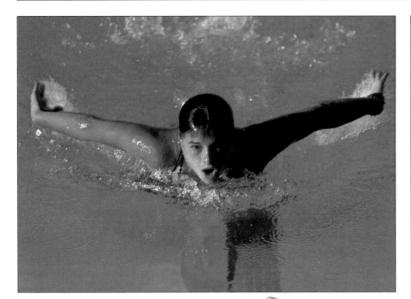

Burning calories
Running, swimming, brisk walking, and bicycling all reduce your body's fat reserves by converting them into energy.

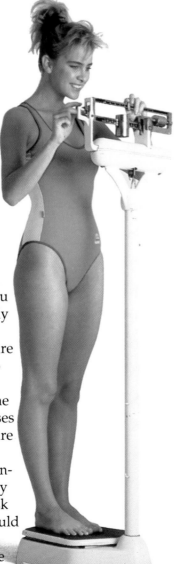

Weight-loss centers
If you find it very difficult to lose weight, it may be helpful to join a weight-loss center, where the discipline of a regular weigh-in and the camaraderie of a shared problem can be a tremendous help. The best organizations employ a balanced, low-calorie diet and behavior modification.

enjoy and that suit your life-style. It is essential that the exercises you choose become a part of your daily activities. Swimming, running, walking, dancing, and bicycling are all good choices. Can you walk to the train or bus every day? Will your schedule allow an hour in the pool several days a week? Exercises that you enjoy are exercises you are more likely to stick with.

Elderly or inactive people can increase their energy expenditure by engaging in activities such as brisk walking. The level of activity should be increased gradually as endurance improves, but care should be taken to stop when fatigue sets in.

ASK YOUR DOCTOR
STAYING TRIM

Q **I have high blood pressure. I am also overweight and have been told to lose weight. Is it true that there's a connection between weight and blood pressure?**

A Yes, there is evidence that excess weight contributes to high blood pressure, which is a risk factor in both heart disease and stroke. You may be able to lower your blood pressure by losing weight.

Q **I have just started taking the birth-control pill and I have noticed that I seem to be putting on weight even though I'm not eating any more than usual. Is weight gain a side effect of the pill?**

A The contraceptive pill can affect women in different ways. There are several different types of pills, some of which may cause fluid retention that leads to weight gain. If you are not happy with your pill, talk to your doctor about it.

Q **I don't eat very much, yet I have difficulty keeping my weight down. Is it true that some people are more prone to being overweight than others?**

A Some fat people do have a particularly slow metabolism, which means that they require relatively little energy from food to keep their bodies running; the extra calories go into weight gain. This is a genetic characteristic, and as such there is nothing you can do about it. You will lose weight if you adjust your diet, but you may have to accept the fact that you have a predisposition to putting on weight and will have to work harder than others to keep weight from accumulating.

MAINTAINING YOUR SKIN AND HAIR

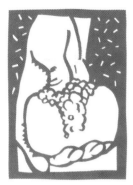

WHEN YOU ARE HEALTHY, your skin and hair generally are too. Eating a balanced diet filled with plenty of fresh fruits and vegetables, drinking at least eight glasses of water every day, and exercising regularly helps keep your skin and hair in good condition from the inside out. However, even the healthiest skin and hair can be compromised by neglect and poor washing.

Knowing your skin, the largest organ in your body, is the first step toward understanding how to care for it. Dry skin is finely textured with few visible pores. It often accompanies a fair complexion and light hair, and tends to burn, flake, and peel easily when exposed to the sun. Oily skin looks shiny, is coarsely textured, and has obvious pores.

SKIN CARE

Men and women can benefit from developing a regular skin care routine, both morning and night, from an early age. Choose skin care products carefully to suit the quality of your skin, but remember that cleansers, cold creams, and

Your facial care routine
Use soap and water to remove any dirt and dead skin that has built up. While your skin is still wet, massage a moisturizer into your face, neck, and throat, concentrating on any area that is particularly dry.

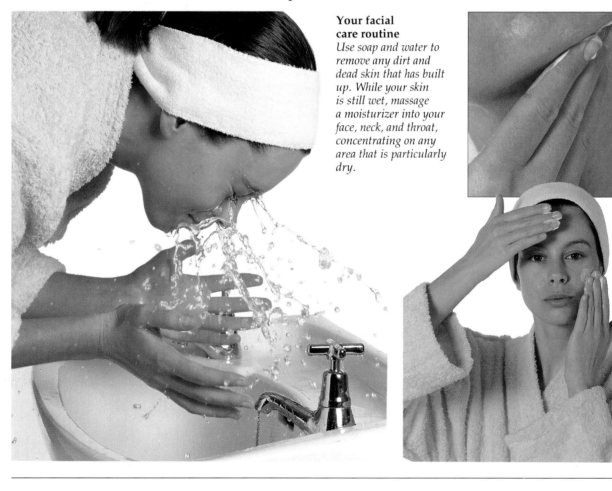

toners are not necessary to maintain a healthy complexion. Water and mild soap are the best tools for keeping normal skin clean. If you have dry skin, wash it with water only. Avoid using very hot water and strong soaps. They can lead to dryness, chapping, and itching. And remember to use enough water to rinse away all traces of soap from your face.

Moisturizing your skin

Moisturizing is probably the most important part of your skin care routine. It helps slow down dehydration of the skin by creating a film on its surface that prevents the natural moisture from escaping. No product can give skin an artificial youthfulness because nothing can penetrate the skin's surface. However, a moisturizer helps keep your skin soft, smooth, and elastic.

Apply moisturizer to wet skin. Massage it in gently and wait a few seconds before removing any excess. The neck and throat can easily become dry, so apply moisturizer there after you wash.

Dealing with blemishes

Pimples and blackheads are the result of the skin pores becoming blocked by oil and dead skin cells. Known as acne, the problem is usually worst at puberty, when hormone levels increase and cause enormous changes in both the size of oil glands in the skin and the amount of oil they produce. The natural oils from your scalp can also cause acne around your hairline and cosmetics that have an oily base may contribute to acne.

Do not be tempted to squeeze your blemishes. This only spreads the bacteria into the lower levels of your skin and can lead to scarring. Instead, ask your doctor to recommend an over-the-counter preparation that you can apply to your skin to help dry up problem areas.

Removing eye makeup
Your eyelashes can become brittle and break off if you leave mascara and other makeup on overnight. Removing your eye makeup before bed also helps prevent your pores from becoming blocked, which can lead to styes.

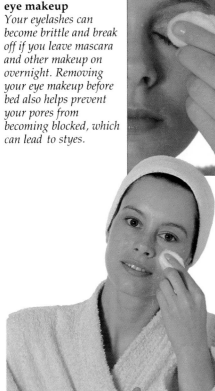

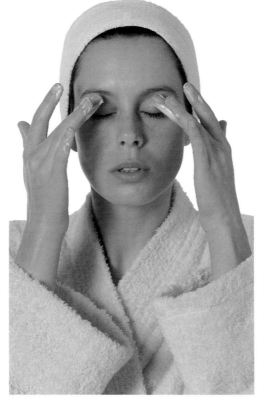

Moisturizing near your eyes
The area of skin around your eyes can be moisturized by applying a cream after every washing.

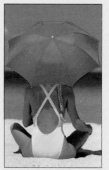

WARNING

Too much exposure to the sun's ultraviolet light can cause sunburn, skin damage, and skin cancer. If you enjoy being in the sun:

♦ Begin with short exposure periods.
♦ Avoid the sun from 10 AM to 2 PM, when the ultraviolet light is most intense.
♦ Use a sunscreen with a high protection factor. To start, use a product with a protection factor of at least 15. Don't wait until you're in the sun before applying a sunscreen; apply it at least 20 to 30 minutes *before* going outside.
♦ Wear sunglasses and a hat.
♦ Be aware that snow and water reflect light and thus increase your exposure to ultraviolet light.
♦ Ensure that your children are adequately protected from the sun by dressing them in T-shirts, hats, and shoes (feet burn easily) and by applying a sunscreen with a high protection factor.

HAND CARE

Your hands take more punishment than any other part of your body, but you can protect them from the worst damage. Wear rubber gloves for cleaning and scrubbing. Sturdy leather gloves will protect your hands when you are working in the yard or around the house. Chapped skin can be prevented by moisturizing your hands regularly. If rubber gloves make your skin red and itchy, wear thin cotton gloves inside them.

Barrier creams also help protect your hands during very dirty work. Always rinse and dry your hands thoroughly afterward, and apply hand cream often, particularly over the knuckles and around the nails. If your hands take a lot of abuse, apply moisturizer and wear a pair of cotton gloves while you sleep.

FOOT CARE

Most people are born with perfect feet, but by the time we reach adulthood four out of five of us have some form of foot trouble. Most problems are caused by lack of regular care and by wearing poorly fitting or high-heeled shoes.

Your feet should be washed every day to minimize the risk of fungal infection. Dry them thoroughly, particularly between the toes. Some people use a hair

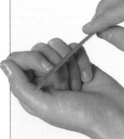

Fingernails
Use an emery board to shape your nails, but leave your cuticles alone. They seal the nail plate and prevent infection from entering. Your nails can be buffed to make them shine.

dryer and talcum powder to help the drying process. When you cut your toenails, always use nail clippers rather than scissors. And remember that cutting your toenails straight across will help prevent painful ingrown toenails.

If you have a problem with foot odor, you may need to wash your feet and change your shoes and socks more often. You can also use an antiperspirant foot spray or talcum powder and deodorized insoles in your shoes.

A good start
Help your child's feet during their primary growth period by providing shoes that fit properly. Buy shoes that leave a little room for growth and don't let your child wear "hand-me-down" shoes from older brothers or sisters.

Foot maintenance
A pumice stone is useful for removing any dead skin from the heels and soles of your feet. Scrubbing with a pumice stone also stimulates blood flow through your feet. After a bath or shower, always dry your feet thoroughly, especially between the toes, to minimize the risk of fungal infection.

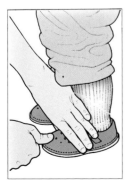

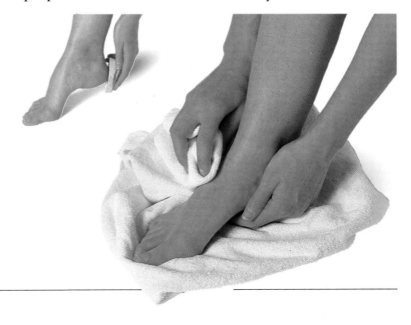

HAIR CARE

The hair root is one of the fastest-growing parts of your body. Hair grows at a rate of about half an inch a month and this growth continues for about 3 years before the hair falls out. A full head of hair consists of between 100,000 and 300,000 hairs. Each of us loses between 100 and 150 hairs a day, some of which are not replaced. The rate at which you lose hair is genetically determined and cannot be altered.

Knowing your hair

Hair tends to fall into one of four categories determined by the amount of oil produced by the sebaceous glands. These glands are located at the top of each hair follicle, close to the surface of the scalp.

Of the four categories of hair, dry hair splits easily, looks dull and brittle, feels rough to the touch, and tangles easily. Oily hair requires frequent washing and is usually associated with oily skin.

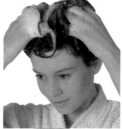

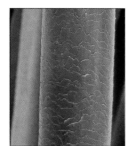

Shampooing
Massage the roots of your hair well. Use the shower stream to rinse your hair thoroughly.

Using a hair dryer
Make sure you hold the dryer at least 6 inches from your hair to avoid heat damage.

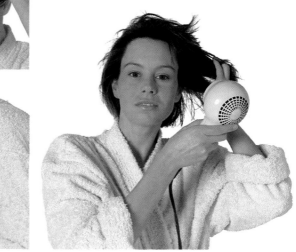

Hair damage
All visible hair is composed of dead cells, but it is still possible to damage it. In healthy hair (right) the outer plates are smooth and lie flat. Damaged hair (below) has a disrupted outer layer with broken and split ends.

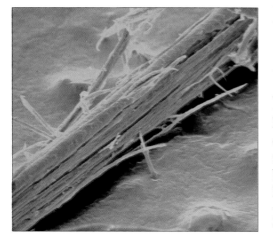

Normal hair has a natural gloss and is smooth and shiny to the touch. If your hair is oily at the scalp and dry at the ends, it is called combination hair.

Washing your hair

Regular washing with a mild shampoo is necessary to remove the buildup of dirt and oil, which form a film on each hair. Dry hair is usually washed every 4 to 6 days; oily hair is washed as often as necessary, sometimes every day. Always rinse your hair thoroughly. Oily hair benefits from a final rinse that contains the strained juice of a lemon.

Using a conditioner smooths the outer surface of the hair. If your hair is oily, apply conditioner only to the ends. If it is dry, comb conditioner through the hair and leave it on for a few minutes before rinsing. Apply more conditioner if you use a hair dryer or a curling iron.

Drying your hair

Hair is at its weakest when wet, and overvigorous rubbing can break and tangle it. After a shower or bath, it is better to wrap your hair in a towel and let it absorb the moisture. Finally, comb your hair with a wide-toothed comb while it is still damp.

BALDNESS

True baldness is very rare in women, but affects 40 percent of men. Women experience a thinning at the temples and over the top of the head from middle age onward. Hair is lost after pregnancy and the menopause, but it returns later.

Male baldness is largely hereditary, beginning at the temples and sides of the forehead and progressing to the crown. There is no cure for baldness, although the drug minoxidil seems to arrest it in some men.

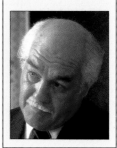

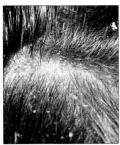

Dandruff
Most dandruff responds quickly to regular washing with one of the many antidandruff shampoos available.

TREATING HAIR PROBLEMS

Most hair problems are caused by harsh hair products, the chemicals used for permanents, and overheating caused by blow-drying, heated rollers, or the sun.

Treating dandruff

Dandruff is a buildup of dead skin cells on the scalp of the head. The condition affects more than 60 percent of the population. The best treatment is to wash your hair regularly with any of the special dandruff shampoos available over the counter. If that is unsuccessful, your doctor can prescribe a shampoo that contains a more powerful ingredient.

Treating split ends

Split ends are a common result of the rough treatment of dry hair. The best solution is to cut off the split ends and then treat the hair. Apply a special deep conditioning treatment before shampooing, then wrap your head in a warm towel for 15 to 30 minutes, changing the towel as necessary. Rinse your hair thoroughly with warm water to remove all the conditioner.

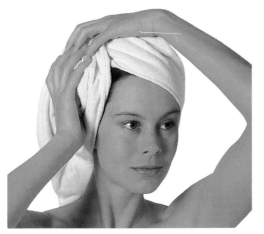

The condition of dry hair can also be improved by applying warm almond or olive oil. After massaging in the oil, wrap your head in a turban for 30 minutes or overnight. To complete the treatment, wash out the oil with shampoo and condition your hair.

GRAY HAIR

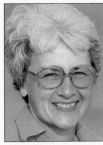

Gray hair is a normal part of aging. Stress, illness, and sudden shock can speed up the graying process. Gray hair is no less healthy than any other hair – it is simply new hair that is growing without any pigment. If you wish to dye your gray hair for cosmetic reasons, try a temporary rinse first or ask a professional to help you.

ASK YOUR DOCTOR CARING FOR YOUR SKIN AND HAIR

Q **I've been reading a lot about Retin-A in the newspaper. What is it, and can it stop me from getting wrinkles?**

A Retin-A (tretinoin) is a derivative of vitamin A that is used for the treatment of acne. It works by peeling off the top layer of the skin and making it swollen, giving it a rosy, smoother look. However, it can also make the skin dry and flaky, increasing the skin's sensitivity to sunlight and irritants. Experts are currently checking the safety of Retin-A because it may stimulate the skin to increase its cell production, which may have implications in the development of skin cancer.

Q **A friend of mine told me that a drug called minoxidil can help stop my baldness. Is this true, and are there any side effects?**

A A twice-daily application of minoxidil does have a positive effect on some men. It is most likely to be effective in young men with early hair loss limited to the crown of the head. Side effects include itchiness and dryness of the scalp. The regrowth of hair ceases when use of the drug is stopped.

Q **I'm thinking about getting my first permanent. Will it damage my hair?**

A A permanent will undoubtedly make your hair much drier; it is not recommended for hair that is already bleached or artificially colored. However, there are some gentler perms available that limit the damage to your hair.

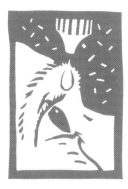

CARING FOR YOUR TEETH AND EYES

Y OUR TEETH AND YOUR EYES are among your most valuable physical assets. In addition to their obvious importance to eating and vision, clean, healthy teeth and bright, clear eyes enhance your appearance and self-confidence.

The second (permanent) teeth you develop as a child are your last natural set, so they require careful attention. Good dental care includes daily brushing and flossing along with regular cleaning and checkups by your dentist.

DENTAL CARE

A few minutes in the morning and evening will help prevent the buildup of plaque, a mixture of food debris and bacteria that is the greatest enemy of teeth and gums. In addition to brushing your teeth at least twice a day, dental floss should be used at least once a day to clean between your teeth. Most people prefer unwaxed floss, but, if you have many fillings or uneven edges, you may prefer waxed floss. When you floss, try not to snap the floss up into your gums. Doing so can damage them.

Dentists sometimes recommend that you massage your gums with rubber stimulator tips to increase gum circulation. However, the stimulators should be used only in addition to regular, thorough brushing and flossing.

BRUSHING YOUR TEETH EFFECTIVELY

Always brush your teeth every morning and evening, and preferably after every meal to remove particles of food, to prevent the buildup of plaque, and to keep your breath fresh. Children's teeth should be brushed as soon as the first teeth appear. Before that, parents should clean children's gums with a piece of damp gauze or with a washcloth.

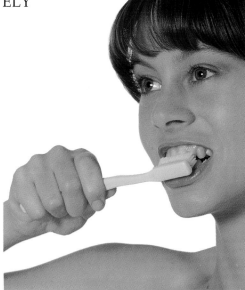

1 Place a soft brush against your teeth at a 45 degree angle, and, using short strokes, gently brush away from the edges of the gum on all sides of each tooth (right). To brush behind the lower front teeth, hold the brush perpendicular to the gum line and use an in-and-out motion.

2 First brush the inside surfaces, then the chewing and outer surfaces of the teeth in the upper jaw.

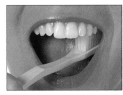

3 Repeat for the teeth in the lower jaw and always rinse your mouth well with water.

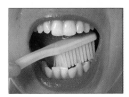

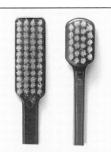

Toothbrush
A brush with soft, rounded bristles is best; harder bristles may damage the tooth enamel and gums. If necessary, use a second brush with a small head to clean the difficult-to-reach areas.

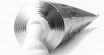

Toothpaste
There is a wide variety of toothpastes on the market. Those containing fluoride are of proven benefit in preventing decay.

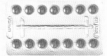

Disclosing agents
These are useful for checking on the efficiency of your brushing. They stain any remaining plaque red.

Using dental floss
Wind the floss around your middle fingers, leaving 4 inches between the two hands. Use a gentle sawing motion to slide the floss between two teeth, then curve the floss into a C- shape against a tooth. Move the floss up and down on the sides of each tooth.

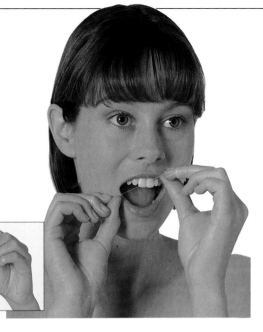

paint stripper. Tobacco smoke also irritates the eyes. The best way to deal with a particle in your eye is explained under FOREIGN BODY IN EYE on page 137.

Avoid rubbing your eyes or eyelids – this is one of the ways in which the eyes can become infected. It is particularly important not to pick at any blemish or cold sore and then touch your eyes.

If your eyes feel sore and tired, tear substitute drops can have a soothing effect, but repeated use is not recommended because it may lead to chronic eye problems. If your eyes continue to feel irritated, dry, or watery, have your doctor examine them (see COMMON EYE AND VISUAL PROBLEMS on pages 96 to 99).

CHOOSING SUNGLASSES

For strong sunlight, sunglasses are recommended because ultraviolet (UV) light can have harmful effects on the eyes. Sunglasses are particularly important during sailing and skiing, due to the UV light reflected off water and snow. High efficiency, UV-blocking sunglasses are worth purchasing. If you wear vision-correcting glasses, you can have them fitted with photochromatic lenses (which darken in strong light), use clip-on filters, or have your prescription made into sunglasses.

Regular checkups

You should visit your dentist twice annually to check for signs of decay and to evaluate the health of your gums. The dentist or hygienist will also scale your teeth and remove any plaque and calculus deposits. Regular checkups are of preventive value as well as a means of addressing problems as they arise.

EYE CARE

Your eyes are delicate, yet remarkably tough and well protected organs. The bones of the skull enclose your eyes in protective sockets, while the eyelids and lashes help keep dust and grit off them. Nevertheless, your eyes require regular care to avoid problems such as irritation, infection, or minor damage, and to keep them looking bright and clear.

Avoiding eye irritation

The outer surface of your eyes can become irritated or damaged by a variety of chemicals. Always wear protective goggles in highly chlorinated swimming pools or when using irritating or dangerous volatile chemicals, such as those contained in some household spray paint, varnish, acid, and

Eye tests

Everyone should have his or her eyes checked periodically – ideally at least every 2 years after the age of 40, though any sudden change in vision should be reported to your doctor or ophthalmologist. Eye tests are particularly important in the very young, when certain problems (such as malaligned eyes) can be corrected before they cause any permanent visual problems or vision loss.

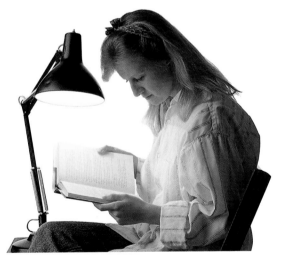

Eye strain
Reading for long periods of time or doing close work in poor light will not damage your eyes but can cause tiredness. Regular headaches when reading may signal the development of a visual problem, which should be checked by your doctor. However, most headaches are not due to an eye disorder.

Contact lenses

Contact lenses have cosmetic appeal, can correct some conditions that glasses cannot, and provide a wider field of vision than glasses. Although many people experience short-term, mild discomfort when they are first fitted with contact lenses, few people are unable to wear them. Contact lenses should always be fitted by a specialist.

Hard lenses are made of a rigid, hard-wearing plastic and provide good crisp vision. Gas-permeable hard lenses, which allow oxygen to reach the surface of the eye, are generally more comfortable but less durable. Soft lenses may be more comfortable than hard lenses, but they are more difficult to maintain.

Extended-wear lenses may be worn for periods of up to 1 month without being removed. They can be useful for the very young and the very old. However, extended-wear lenses need careful sterilization and professional supervision because they carry a much greater risk of complications, such as infection.

USING CONTACT LENSES SAFELY

1 Always wash your hands thoroughly before inserting lenses to prevent introducing an infection into your eyes.

2 Store and clean your lenses meticulously, using the special solutions recommended for your type of lenses.

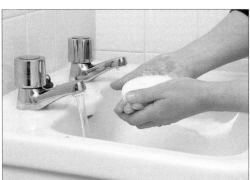

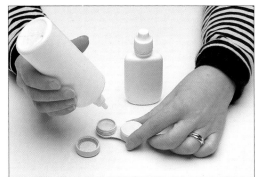

3 If any discomfort or redness develops, remove the lens from your eye immediately.

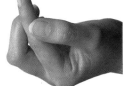

ASK YOUR DOCTOR EYE CARE

Q I'm 35 and have been wearing contact lenses since I was 20. Will there be a time when I'll no longer be able to wear them?

A Probably not. Many hard lens wearers develop an intolerance, with discomfort and shorter wearing times, after years of satisfactory wear, but the problem can often be solved by switching to gas-permeable or soft lenses. Soft-lens wearers sometimes become allergic to solutions containing preservatives.

Q I wear a lot of eye makeup and I've heard that this can be bad for my eyes. Is this true?

A Eye makeup usually does not affect vision. Any bad effects – which are rare – are generally confined to the lid or the conjunctiva lining the lids, and are usually caused by irritation or allergy. The continual application and removal of eye makeup may, however, stretch the skin around your eyes.

Q Can staring at a computer screen or a television for several hours harm my eyes?

A There is no evidence that either of these activities has any harmful effect. However, staring at a computer screen or TV for hours at a time may put a strain on some of the muscles around your eyes (particularly if you have a tendency to squint, which could mean you need your eyes tested or a new prescription for your glasses). Hours of viewing may result in a feeling of tiredness around the eyes and discomfort often referred to as "eye strain." To help avoid this strain, take short breaks in your work or TV viewing.

CHAPTER FOUR

PRACTICAL HOME NURSING

INTRODUCTION

MAKING YOUR
PATIENT
COMFORTABLE

TENDING TO YOUR
PATIENT'S NEEDS

ALL FAMILIES know the challenges involved in taking care of a parent or child who is affected by a long-term illness or who is confined to bed temporarily. Whether the patient has been in the hospital for surgery or is recovering from an accident, the day he or she returns home can be highly stressful for the family. Much of this anxiety can be eliminated, however, if the family plans in advance for the patient's return. Preparing the patient's room and equipping it with some forethought and imagination goes a long way toward creating an atmosphere of calm and cheerfulness that is conducive to recovery.

Nursing a patient through convalescence at home requires a keen appreciation of his or her needs. You may want to ask yourself "How would I want to be cared for if I were ill?" Your patient's needs are most acute when he or she is immobile and thus reliant on the family for the most basic functions. He or she may require help in eating, elimination, bathing, and staying warm and comfortable in bed. Some of these tasks require special techniques that should be learned to ensure the safety of the patient. In addition, there are measures that can help prevent medical complications or setbacks. For example,

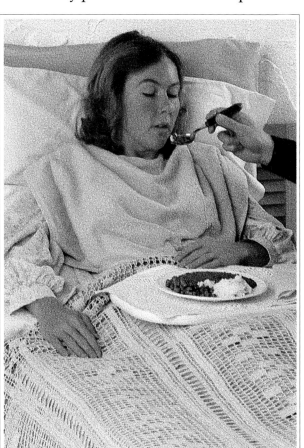

a patient with a heart condition who has recently been discharged from the hospital should not be subjected to too much stress or be allowed to exercise beyond reasonable limits. And with any patient who is confined to bed long-term, preventing bedsores is always a major consideration. The family also needs to be aware of the patient's psychological requirements. High morale is a positive influence upon the individual recovering from illness and injury. You can maintain the patient's self-esteem by encouraging him or her to do as much as possible unaided, and gradually to regain any independence he or she may have lost during the illness. In some cases following a serious illness or accident, some simple skills have to be relearned from scratch. Mental stimulation, companionship, and communication with others all help to hasten the recovery process. Visitors should be welcomed, but only if they don't exhaust your recovering family member. Try to assess his or her condition to decide how much visiting is advisable, and discuss your opinion with the family. At the same time, the family must remember that the patient may be feeling vulnerable. Helping the patient should be done with an awareness of his or her need for privacy and a proper respect for dignity.

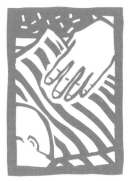

MAKING YOUR PATIENT COMFORTABLE

A PERSON WHO IS recovering from illness, injury, or surgery may need to spend many hours each day resting in bed. As a nurse, your first task is to ensure that the patient is as comfortable as possible. Even if your patient is mobile, he or she may still need assistance when sitting up, when getting in and out of bed, or when using the bathroom.

Few people are accustomed to spending entire days, weeks, or months in bed, and a helpless and unattended patient can find convalescence an ordeal of tedium, pain, and discomfort. A sympathetic caregiver can do much to make the experience tolerable, but he or she must be aware of using the correct procedures. Moving a helpless patient can be difficult, and it is important that you put neither the patient nor yourself under any unnecessary strain.

CARING FOR AN IMMOBILE PATIENT

A bedridden person may be immobile because he or she is unconscious for long periods or because a physical disability impedes his or her movement. Caring for such patients may involve moving them yourself. Before you do so, however, ask the doctor whether moving the patient is advisable.

CHANGING A BED WITHOUT MOVING THE PATIENT

Two people are needed to carry out this procedure. The patient should be told that you need to roll him or her over in the bed. Make sure the room is warm and that you have laid out the clean linen nearby. A laundry basket for holding the soiled linen is also helpful.

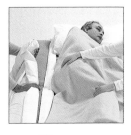

2 Support the patient while your helper tucks in the new bottom sheet and unrolls it toward the patient's back.

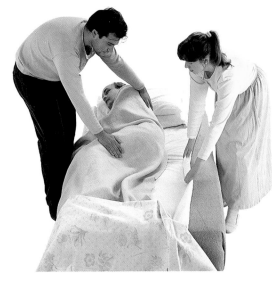

1 Remove the bedspread and all but one blanket, putting them aside in the order you will want to replace them. Also remove the top sheet. Keep the patient covered with one blanket to prevent chilling. Then roll the patient toward you and support him or her on one side of the bed, as shown, by holding his or her back and thigh. Your helper then untucks and rolls up the soiled bottom sheet.

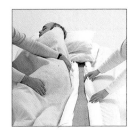

3 Your helper rolls the patient over the ridge of sheets onto the newly laid clean side, supporting him or her while you remove the soiled sheet and tuck in the clean bottom sheet.

4 Put on the new top sheet, replace the blanket and bedspread, and change the pillowcases. You may want to change the patient's pajamas, being sure you keep him or her warm.

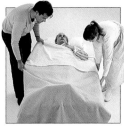

Bedsores

Bedsores are breaks in the skin produced by pressure. They frequently develop in people who are bedridden and cannot move easily or who lack normal skin sensation. The sores, also called pressure sores and decubitus ulcers, are common in stroke patients and in people with back injuries. Bedsores form when the weight of the body cuts off circulation to areas that are in contact with the bed. The affected tissues, deprived of oxygen, become red and eventually die, giving way to open wounds. The most common sites for bedsores are the heels, hips, buttocks, elbows, shoulders, and back of the head.

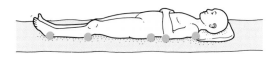

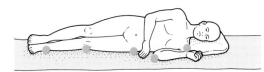

Sites of bedsores
Shown in pink are the parts of the body most vulnerable to pressure in a patient who is sitting or lying for long periods of time.

To prevent bedsores in an immobile patient, turn him or her every 2 hours, being careful not to produce any friction on the skin. The skin should be kept clean and dry and lubricated with a body cream or lotion to give added protection. If the patient is incontinent, it is important to keep the skin, clothing, and linen as dry as possible.

Diet should contain adequate fluids, protein, and vitamins. A nurse can show you how to massage the skin and joints of vulnerable areas. In addition, keep the bottom bedsheet taut and remove any loose items such as tissue or food crumbs. Natural or artificial sheepskin protectors can be purchased to relieve pressure on the hips, knees, and heels. Special air mattresses are also available.

SITTING THE PATIENT UP IN BED

For a patient who is confined to bed, sitting up with firm support can relieve soreness from pressure points. It is safest for two people to lift the patient's weight, but one person can do it without risk if the correct technique is used.

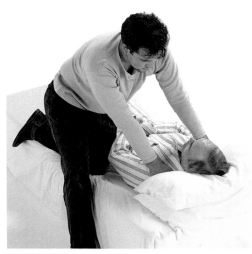

1 First, arrange pillows or a backrest to elevate the patient's shoulders. Cross the patient's arms, resting them at his or her waist. Place your hands over the patient's shoulders and the inner part of your knee on the bed adjacent to the patient's hip. Have your other foot on the floor slightly ahead of your opposite knee and in line with the patient's waist.

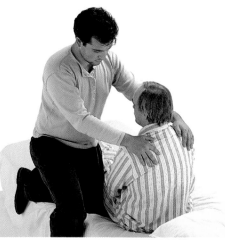

2 Make sure your hands are securely placed on his or her shoulders, so that you will be able to support the patient after you sit him or her up. Your own weight will raise the patient as you sit back, keeping your arms straight and drawing the patient up toward your body.

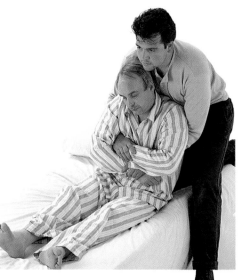

3 If it is necessary to move the patient up in the bed, have the patient cross his or her arms. With the inner part of your knee behind the patient and your weight on your other foot, hold the patient's forearms from behind as shown. Sit back and your weight will pull him or her up.

PLANNING THE SICKROOM

When people are ill or disabled, their movements are usually restricted and they may be confined to one room for an extended time. The morale of your patient can be greatly affected by his or her physical surroundings, so it is essential to select, equip, and organize a room with attention to detail.

A sink nearby is useful for filling water pitchers, wiping up spills, and bathing the bedridden patient.

An angled light firmly clamped to the head of the bed may be more easily controlled than a bedside lamp.

The bedside table should be tall enough to enable the patient to reach it without straining. Some people require many items near them, including a water pitcher and drinking glass, medications, reading material, tissues, clock, radio, telephone, TV remote control, and whistle or bell to call for assistance.
If your patient is young or confused, keep all medications away from the bedside.

A hot-water bottle or an electric heating pad can be used for comfort from chills or aches. These heating devices are not suitable for babies or for the confused or paralyzed patient. Secondary skin burns are possible if hot-water bottles and heating pads are used incorrectly for extended periods.

The bed should have a firm mattress with access to both sides to facilitate changing the bed and washing the patient. If long-term care at home is anticipated, you may want to consider renting a hospital bed.

A bed tray is convenient for serving meals and providing a firm surface for cards, puzzles, and games.

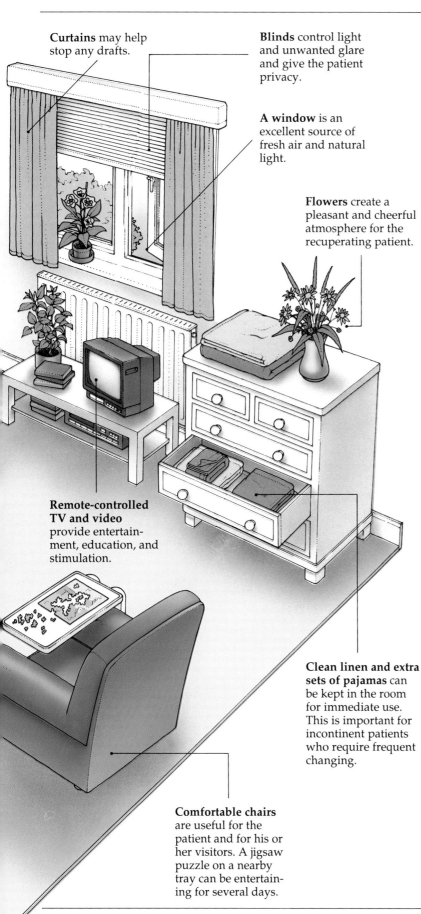

Curtains may help stop any drafts.

Blinds control light and unwanted glare and give the patient privacy.

A window is an excellent source of fresh air and natural light.

Flowers create a pleasant and cheerful atmosphere for the recuperating patient.

Remote-controlled TV and video provide entertainment, education, and stimulation.

Clean linen and extra sets of pajamas can be kept in the room for immediate use. This is important for incontinent patients who require frequent changing.

Comfortable chairs are useful for the patient and for his or her visitors. A jigsaw puzzle on a nearby tray can be entertaining for several days.

A COMFORTABLE ENVIRONMENT

A patient's room should be cheerful, well lit, reasonably quiet, uncluttered, comfortably warm, well ventilated, and close to a bathroom. The room should be as clean as possible, especially if the patient has any wound or burned area of skin that is susceptible to infection. Most people prefer to be cared for in their own bedrooms when they are ill. However, if the bedroom in question lacks the comforts mentioned previously, locate a more suitable environment. Even the living room, if it can be kept free of distraction, can be set up with a hospital bed (rented, if necessary) and other amenities.

Comfort in bed

People recovering from illness or injury can be helped by simple but comfortable supports in bed. These include backrests and triangular pillows for those who sit up for long periods and have the potential to develop backaches. Orthopedic bed boards can be placed under a soft mattress, giving support to people with back problems. A pillow wrapped in a sheet can act as a footrest. In addition, it can be used to keep the weight of the sheet and blanket off the feet of a patient who has suffered a stroke, wound, or burn in the lower body or legs.

Mental stimulation

As the condition of your patient improves, mental stimulation becomes an increasingly important factor in the recovery process. Children should be read to and given books, toys, and creative projects that involve their attention, such as coloring books and crayons or modeling clay. Adults will enjoy their favorite magazines, newspapers, videotapes, and television programs. Books recorded on audiotapes are entertaining for people who don't have the energy to sit up to read or watch television.

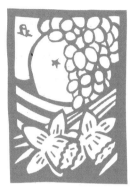

TENDING TO YOUR PATIENT'S NEEDS

WHEN CARING FOR someone at home, you will find it useful to establish a daily routine to keep your patient clean and comfortable. Find out how much help the patient requires to perform essential tasks and allow him or her to attend to personal needs as much as possible. This helps maintain the person's self-esteem, and makes him or her feel less dependent.

The amount of assistance a convalescent needs during the day varies with the individual. People who are not seriously ill or disabled may be able to attend to personal hygiene on their own. However, changing linen, preparing meals, shopping for groceries, and doing the laundry requires more energy. If you are caring for someone during a long illness, you may need to help the patient bathe, eat regular meals, use the toilet, or get out of bed for a short walk.

WASHING AND BATHING

Although it is important for a convalescent to stay clean for hygienic reasons, bathing also refreshes anyone who is ill. Encourage your patient to bathe daily by helping him or her to the bathroom or by providing washing equipment at the bedside. If your patient cannot bathe on his or her own, you may need to give a bed bath, as shown below.

GIVING A BED BATH

1 Wash and dry one area of the body at a time, working from the head toward the feet. Uncover only the part you are washing, so that the patient does not become chilled. Many patients are able to wash their own genital regions, but changing the water is necessary if you plan to wash other parts of the body.

2 When you have washed the front of the person's body, roll him or her over to one side so that you can reach the back. Help the person into fresh clothing if his or her clothes are sweaty or soiled.

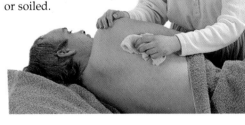

3 When drying your patient's body, pat his or her skin gently with a towel. A light dusting of talcum powder helps the skin remain dry and gives a clean, fresh feeling.

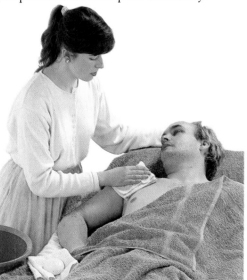

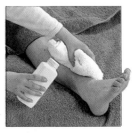

EQUIPMENT FOR A BED BATH

You will need the following:
♦ A mild, unperfumed soap to avoid irritation
♦ A basin of hot water
♦ Two washcloths – one for the face and body and one for the genital area
♦ Two towels for drying these areas
♦ Two large bath towels – one to keep the convalescent warm and one to protect the bedding
♦ Talcum powder to freshen the patient

Helping with personal care

It is important to help convalescents take care of their teeth, eyes, and hair. Teeth should be brushed twice daily by the patient or by you. If dried tears have formed crusts in the corners of the patient's eyes, gently wipe the crusts away with a warm, moistened washcloth.

Many people feel more comfortable during an illness if their hair is washed regularly. To wash the hair in bed, lean the patient's head over a bowl on the floor, making sure that his or her neck is well supported by the edge of the bed. Use a bottle of water to wet the hair, and thoroughly rinse it after shampooing. If the patient cannot be moved, wash the hair with a no-rinse shampoo.

FEEDING AND ELIMINATION

An important part of your daily routine involves feeding the patient and helping him or her use the bathroom. Some people may feel embarrassed, so try to be as sympathetic as possible.

Preparing meals

Some people want only bland foods when they feel ill, but even scrambled eggs and toast can be made more appealing with the addition of an orange slice and some parsley. If you are preparing the meals, a little extra effort will help your patient look forward to mealtimes and eat the variety of foods you offer. If no special diet is necessary, the sick person can eat the same types of food he or she normally would.

Assisting at mealtime

Unless they are seriously ill, people recovering at home usually prefer to feed themselves. Make sure that your patient sits up straight and that he or she is well supported by pillows to promote a safe posture for swallowing. If you are caring for a helpless person, consult a nurse about special feeding techniques.

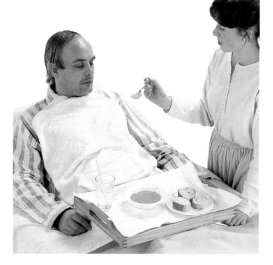

Feeding a helpless person
Talk to the disabled person while you are spoon-feeding him or her. Don't expect replies throughout the meal, however; the effort of swallowing may make the person tired. Allow plenty of time for food to be chewed and swallowed between mouthfuls.

Dealing with excretions

When your patient needs to urinate or move his or her bowels, be conscious of the need for privacy. A mobile person should be helped to the bathroom when necessary. A less mobile patient may be lifted onto a portable toilet placed beside the bed. If the patient is not mobile, use a bedpan or urinal.

Helping your patient use the portable toilet or bedpan at the same time each day can encourage regulation of his or her bowel action.

Using a bedpan
Warm the pan with hot water and dry it thoroughly before use. Help the patient raise his or her buttocks with one hand, and slip the bedpan underneath with the other. This procedure may be easier with the person sitting upright, if this is possible. Never leave the pan in position longer than necessary; the pressure can cause bedsores.

CHAPTER FIVE

BASIC FIRST AID

INTRODUCTION

DEALING WITH MAJOR EMERGENCIES

A-Z OF HOME FIRST AID

ACCIDENTS ARE the leading cause of death and disability up to the age of 44. If anything, economic growth and greater leisure time appear to be increasing the hazards. For example, the number of people using motor vehicles is increasing, as is the use of electrical equipment in the home. Fortunately, most accidental injuries are minor and require only basic first aid. However, the ability to cope with a life-threatening emergency is invaluable and can mean the difference between life and death. When an accident victim has only minutes to live, the first person on the scene must be able to take immediate and appropriate first-aid action.

The information in this chapter is designed to help you deal effectively with both minor and serious accidents involving others or yourself. The chapter is divided into two sections. The first part, DEALING WITH MAJOR EMERGENCIES, provides instructions to help you respond safely in an emergency situation. The illustrated, step-by-step sequences help you determine your responsibilities as a provider of first aid. In some circumstances, the goal of initial first aid is to prevent an illness or injury from getting any worse, to summon the help of a doctor, paramedic, or other trained medical person, and to reassure the accident victim. When medical aid cannot be obtained, the correct use of lifesaving techniques may be necessary to stop severe bleeding or restore breathing. The second section, A-Z OF HOME FIRST AID, outlines the treatment of common minor injuries, such as cuts, bruises, and nosebleeds, that often occur in or around the home. Also included are measures to improve home safety and an illustrated list of items you should keep in your home first-aid kit. Some of the illnesses and injuries covered in this section require only basic first aid unless problems develop. However, the section explains clearly when you should seek medical help.

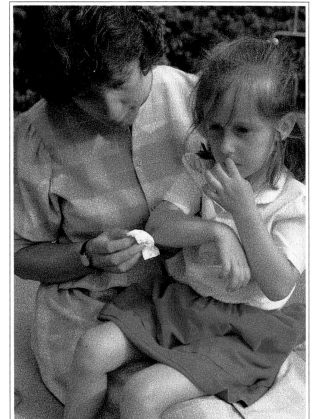

By familiarizing yourself with the basic first-aid techniques described in this book, you will be better prepared for an emergency. However, formal training is recommended to learn proper lifesaving measures, such as cardiopulmonary resuscitation (CPR) and the Heimlich maneuver. No book can substitute for the experience you can gain from a first-aid class. In fact, CPR should only be attempted if you have detailed written instructions to follow or have been trained in the technique. For information, contact your local heart association or the American National Red Cross.

DEALING WITH MAJOR EMERGENCIES

If you are faced with an emergency situation, you should give what first aid you can on the spot. While you are giving emergency treatment, send someone else to get professional help or call out for assistance. Determine if the victim is breathing and if his or her heart is beating (see below and opposite). Make the victim as comfortable as possible and treat any signs of shock (see page 132).

In some cases, the quickest way to get medical help is to drive the person yourself to the nearest hospital. However, do not attempt to move the patient on your own if you suspect a back injury or if the victim is highly distressed or unconscious. Remember that you must move the victim if you and he or she are in imminent danger – near fire, poisonous fumes, a potential explosion, a collapsing building, and so on.

EMERGENCY CHECKLIST

1 First determine if the victim is breathing. If the victim is not breathing, begin ARTIFICIAL RESUSCITATION (opposite page).

2 If the victim does not respond, check his or her heartbeat. If you cannot detect a heartbeat or pulse at the wrist or neck, begin CARDIOPULMONARY RESUSCITATION (below) if you are familiar with the technique.

3 Control any SEVERE BLEEDING (see page 133).

4 Treat any SEVERE BURNS (see page 133).

5 Watch for signs of SHOCK (see page 132).

HEART STOPPAGE

If someone's heart has stopped beating, it can sometimes be revived by cardiopulmonary resuscitation (CPR), which consists of chest compressions performed in conjunction with artificial resuscitation.

Before giving CPR, you must determine if the victim's heart has stopped beating. The person will be unresponsive, skin color will be gray, no pulse will be felt at the wrist or neck, and no heartbeat will be audible in the chest. If someone is breathing, then the heart *is* beating, even if you cannot feel a pulse.

CARDIOPULMONARY RESUSCITATION

1 First make sure that the airway is clear. Then look, listen, and feel for signs of breathing.

2 If the victim is breathing, make sure that he or she is comfortable and call out for someone to get help. Stay with the victim.

3 If the victim is not breathing, administer ARTIFICIAL RESUSCITATION (opposite page).

4 If your attempts at restarting breathing fail and you cannot detect a pulse or heartbeat, start chest compressions. Place the heel of one hand on the lower third of the breastbone and cover with the heel of the other hand. Push down forcefully but smoothly about 1.5 to 2 inches without bending your elbows. Release pressure with each compression to allow the chest to expand.

5 Repeat step 4 at the rate of 80 compressions every minute, giving two breaths by artificial resuscitation after every 15 compressions.

6 As soon as you detect a pulse or heartbeat, resume artificial resuscitation and continue until the victim is breathing on his or her own.

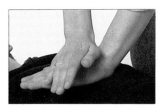

WARNING

Do not attempt to carry out cardiopulmonary resuscitation unless you have succinct written instructions or have been thoroughly trained in the technique. The information at left briefly explains CPR basics.

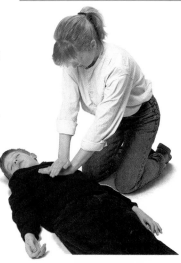

130

WEAK OR ABSENT BREATHING

If you come upon an individual whose breathing is weak, shallow, or labored, stay with the victim and call out for someone to get help.

If the individual is not breathing, there will be no noticeable up and down movement of the chest or abdomen and the skin color will become blue-gray. Most importantly, you will not *hear* or *feel* air being exhaled by the victim. If you are in doubt about whether the victim is or is not breathing, kneel down very close to him or her and turn your head so that your ear is just above the victim's mouth and nose. If the victim is breathing, you will *hear* air being exhaled and you will *feel* his or her breath on your ear. If the victim is *not* breathing, you must breathe artificially for him or her by breathing directly into the lungs, using either the mouth-to-mouth or mouth-to-nose method.

Mouth-to-nose resuscitation

If the victim has a facial injury that makes it difficult to breathe into his or her mouth, use the mouth-to-nose method. First, tilt the victim's head backward using the palm of your hand. With the fingers of your other hand, close the victim's mouth by lifting the chin. Take a deep breath, seal your mouth around the victim's nose, and blow into the nose. Remove your mouth and hold the victim's mouth open so that air can escape. Repeat every 5 seconds.

ARTIFICIAL RESUSCITATION: MOUTH-TO-MOUTH

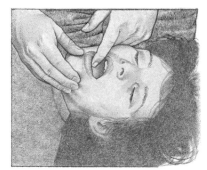

1 Quickly clear the mouth and airway of any foreign material with your fingers. Loosen any clothing around the victim's neck and chest.

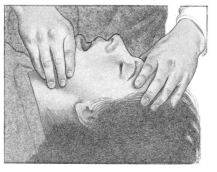

2 To open the victim's airway, tilt his or her head backward by placing one hand on the forehead and then placing the fingers of your other hand under the bony part of his or her chin.

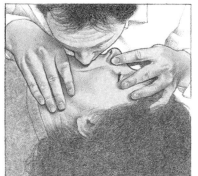

3 Using the hand that is placed on the victim's forehead, pinch the nostrils closed. Take a deep breath, seal your mouth over the victim's mouth, and exhale. Turn to watch the victim's chest rise. Stop blowing when the chest expands.

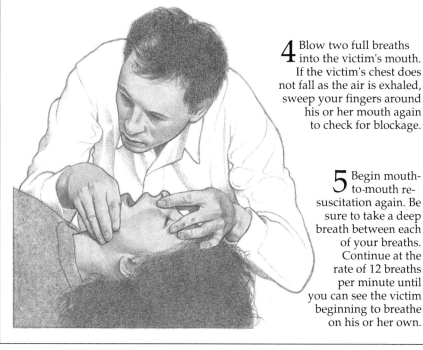

4 Blow two full breaths into the victim's mouth. If the victim's chest does not fall as the air is exhaled, sweep your fingers around his or her mouth again to check for blockage.

5 Begin mouth-to-mouth resuscitation again. Be sure to take a deep breath between each of your breaths. Continue at the rate of 12 breaths per minute until you can see the victim beginning to breathe on his or her own.

RESUSCITATING A BABY OR SMALL CHILD

Seal your mouth over the mouth and nose. Do not tip the head back very far because you may close off the airway. Blow gently into the lungs, at the rate of one breath every 2 to 3 seconds.

SHOCK

Any severe injury can lead to shock, particularly if there are severe burns or bleeding. First-aid treatment following all severe injuries should include measures to prevent, or at least minimize, shock.

A person who is in shock usually feels faint and is pale and sweaty, with a weak, rapid pulse and cold, clammy skin. He or she may also be thirsty and may gradually become drowsy. Eventually, he or she may lose consciousness.

How to help prevent shock

1 Lay the victim down and raise the legs (unless there is a fracture).

2 Loosen any tight clothing and prevent heat loss by wrapping the victim in a coat or blanket. Do not try to restore heat by using an electric blanket or hot-water bottle.

3 Make the victim as comfortable as possible and offer reassurance. Do not give him or her anything to eat or drink.

ELECTRIC SHOCK

Severe electric shock can knock a person to the ground, cause unconsciousness, and even stop the victim from breathing and the heart from beating. Although you may see only a small burn mark on the skin, there may be widespread internal damage. A person who has experienced severe electric shock should always be examined by a doctor.

What to do

1 Turn off the current, if possible, or push the victim away from the electricity source with a dry, noncon-
ducting object such as a broom. Until you have done this, the victim may continue to conduct electricity and you may receive a substantial shock if you touch him or her.

2 Check the victim's breathing. If breathing has stopped, start ARTIFICIAL RESUSCITATION (page 131) immediately. You may have to continue for up to 30 minutes before the victim's normal breathing resumes.

3 If the victim does not begin breathing on his or her own after five breaths, check the pulse at the neck or at the wrist. If there is none, CARDIOPULMONARY RESUSCITATION (page 130) may also be needed.

4 When the victim is breathing again, treat any visible SEVERE BURNS (opposite page) and call for medical help. Stay with the victim.

DROWNING

In a drowning accident, it is vital to start ARTIFICIAL RESUSCITATION (page 131) immediately if the victim is not breathing. Call out for assistance and move the victim to a hard surface (e.g., a pier, a boat, or the shore) as quickly as you can.

If the victim is in shallow water, attempt to restore breathing in the water; then move the victim to safety. Keep him or her warm with clothes or blankets, and call out again for someone to get medical help. Stay with the victim. (Water life-saving classes to ensure your own safety and the safety of the victim are recommended.)

POISONING

Accidental poisoning, usually by swallowing liquid cleaning solutions or other poisons, is one of the most common accidents in the home. Young children are in particular danger. All poisonous substances (including alcoholic beverages and prescription and over-the-counter drugs) should be kept well out of reach of children.

What to do

1 If the victim is conscious, ask what he or she has swallowed. Then call immediately for an ambulance and tell the paramedics on the phone what the victim has taken.

2 If the person is conscious and you are certain that corrosives have not been swallowed, induce vomiting by giving ipecac or sticking your fingers down the person's throat.

3 If the victim is not breathing, start ARTIFICIAL RESUSCITATION (page 131) immediately. Use the mouth-to-nose method to avoid contact with a corrosive poison.

4 If the victim is unconscious but breathing, or conscious but drowsy, ensure that he or she is comfortable and call out for someone to get professional help. Stay with the victim and provide reassurance.

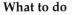

BLEEDING

Bleeding that cannot be stopped easily after a few minutes of direct pressure (or a wound that spurts blood forcefully) is an emergency. Severe blood loss can lead to shock, unconsciousness, and death. It is essential to stem the flow of blood quickly and efficiently.

How to stop severe bleeding

1 Lay the victim down and, if possible, raise the injured part above the level of the heart.

2 Remove any visible and easily accessible foreign bodies such as pieces of glass, but do not probe for anything that is deeply embedded.

3 Press hard on the wound with a clean pad, holding the edges of the wound together. If there is still a foreign body in the wound, press around it, not over it.

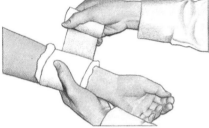

4 Maintain pressure by binding a clean bandage around the pad.

5 If blood oozes through, do not remove the first dressing but put other dressings on top of the first and bandage firmly to hold in place.

SEVERE BURNS

Burns may be caused by dry heat, such as fire; by moist heat, such as hot liquids and steam; or by electricity, corrosive chemicals, or friction.

The severity of a burn depends partly on the percentage of body area affected and partly on the depth of the burn. A first-degree burn injures only the outside layer of the skin. Second-degree burns damage the layers beneath the surface. The deepest type, a third-degree burn, destroys all layers of skin, leaving a painless white or charred area.

CHOKING

If an object blocks the airway so that coughing and breathing are difficult or impossible, emergency first aid such as the Heimlich maneuver (right) is needed. In adults, the obstruction is usually a fish bone or a piece of meat. In children, who have much narrower airways, the obstruction may be a peanut or a small toy.

If the victim is unconscious:

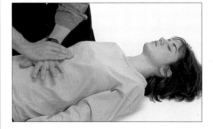

1 Place the heel of one hand against the middle of the patient's abdomen, slightly above the navel. Place your other hand on top and press down and upward toward the head with a quick thrust. Repeat if needed.

How to revive a choking baby

1 Support the baby along the length of your arm, stabilizing the head by supporting the baby's jaw.

2 Give several gentle thumps between the shoulder blades with the heel of your hand. If these efforts do not work, turn the baby over and give four quick chest thrusts.

If the victim is conscious:

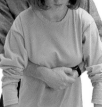

1 Grasp the victim from behind with one fist placed under the breastbone, with the thumb side in, and the other hand holding the fist.

2 Make a quick, thrusting movement, inward and upward. Repeat if necessary.

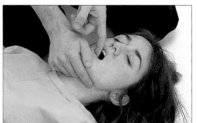

2 If your efforts fail, tilt the head back, open the mouth, and try to remove the object with your finger. If breathing stops, carry out ARTIFICIAL RESUSCITATION (page 131) and call for emergency help.

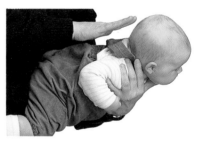

How to deal with severe burns

1 If a person's clothes are on fire, smother the flames with whatever is on hand (not plastic) or roll the victim back and forth on the ground. Call for help immediately.

2 Remove any clothing that has been soaked in hot fat, boiling water, or corrosive chemicals, but do not remove any dry, burned clothing that has stuck to the skin over the burn.

3 Do not apply lotions or ointments. Cover any exposed burned areas with a clean, nonfluffy pad (such as a sheet) to prevent infection.

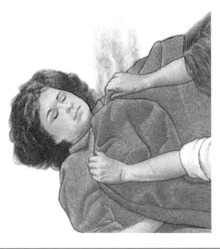

A-Z OF HOME FIRST AID

Minor injuries are common occurrences in and around the home. You can treat most home accidents yourself (see BASIC HOME FIRST-AID KIT below), but it is also important to know when you should seek medical help. This section provides you with quick access to information that will enable you to cope with most everyday accidents.

Safety in the home
You can do much to prevent accidental injury in and around the home by following the basic safety precautions listed at right.

SAFETY CHECKLIST

1 Keep all medicines and poisonous substances out of reach of children.

2 Check electrical wiring and equipment regularly to make sure it is not faulty.

3 Keep all sharp implements in drawers and always face any pan handles inward on the stove.

4 Guard against falls by ensuring rugs are nonslip, there are no trailing wires, and stairs are well lit.

BASIC HOME FIRST-AID KIT

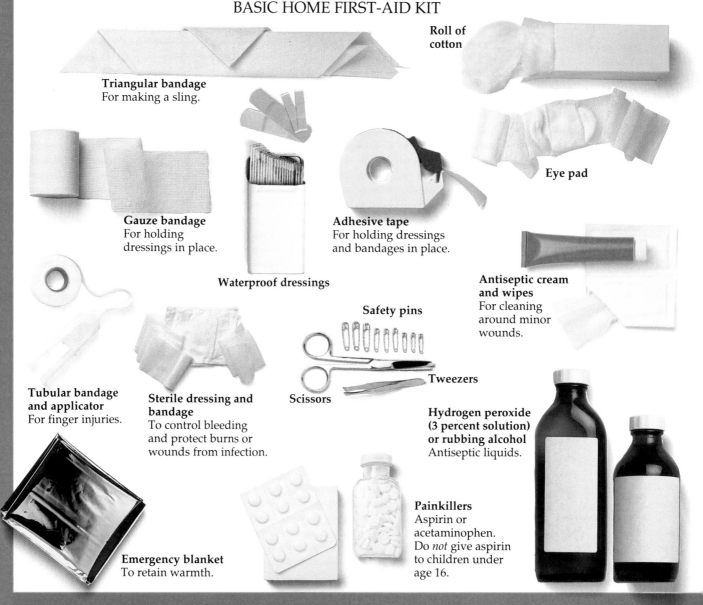

Triangular bandage
For making a sling.

Roll of cotton

Eye pad

Gauze bandage
For holding dressings in place.

Adhesive tape
For holding dressings and bandages in place.

Waterproof dressings

Antiseptic cream and wipes
For cleaning around minor wounds.

Safety pins

Tubular bandage and applicator
For finger injuries.

Sterile dressing and bandage
To control bleeding and protect burns or wounds from infection.

Scissors

Tweezers

Hydrogen peroxide (3 percent solution) or rubbing alcohol
Antiseptic liquids.

Painkillers
Aspirin or acetaminophen. Do *not* give aspirin to children under age 16.

Emergency blanket
To retain warmth.

BITES AND STINGS

Many different mammals, insects, snakes, and other animals are capable of inflicting injury through biting or stinging. Each type of injury requires slightly different first-aid treatment.

MAMMAL BITES

Any mammal bite, whether from a domestic pet (such as a dog), a wild animal (such as a skunk), or a human, requires medical attention. The bite may become infected if not treated promptly and may also carry the risk of tetanus and rabies.

INSECT STINGS

A relatively small number of insects, including wasps, bees, hornets, and yellow jackets, are capable of stinging. Stings cause pain, redness, and swelling that last for about 48 hours. Although it normally takes a large number of insect stings – usually hundreds in the case of an adult – to be life-threatening, about one person in 200 is allergic to insect venom. An allergic reaction to a sting can cause dizziness, facial swelling, an itchy rash, wheezing, and vomiting, and can lead to SHOCK (page 132). This type of severe reaction, called anaphylactic shock, usually occurs only in people who have been stung on a previous occasion and have become hypersensitive.

How to treat a sting

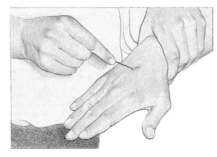

1 Remove any stinger left in the skin by gently scraping it out with a knife blade or needle. Do not pull on it with your fingers or squeeze it with tweezers. This can squeeze more venom into the wound.

2 Wash the stung area with soap and water and apply hydrocortisone cream or a weak solution of ammonia to counteract the acidity of the sting.

3 Apply a cold compress or ice pack to help reduce swelling. If the symptoms of anaphylactic shock develop, treat the victim for shock and get medical help immediately.

4 A sting in the mouth can be dangerous because swelling may interfere with breathing. Seek medical help immediately and give the victim ice cubes to suck.

SNAKE BITES

About 45,000 people are bitten by snakes in the US each year, but the number of deaths is less than 20. This is partly because the majority of bites are received from nonpoisonous species. In addition, most poisonous snakebites can be treated effectively if the victim can be moved to a hospital quickly.

How to treat a snakebite

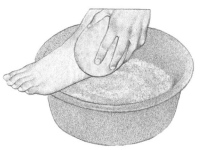

1 Wash around the wound with soap and water and give a mild analgesic.

2 Immobilize the bitten part and keep the victim still. Do not raise the injured limb.

3 If the victim is pale or sweating, feels faint, or has difficulty breathing, lay the victim down, and keep him or her warm.

4 If the victim is nauseous, turn the victim on his or her side so that any secretions can drain out. Get medical help.

BLISTERS

Blisters on the skin may be the result of an allergic reaction or may occur from friction, burns, or chemicals. No first aid is needed unless the blister breaks or is located in an area where it will be irritated by friction. In these instances, wash the area with soap and water and cover with an adhesive bandage. Never deliberately break a blister. Doing so leaves a raw area of skin that may become infected. If a blister looks infected, consult your doctor.

BRUISING

A bruise occurs when a blow or fall causes bleeding into the tissues beneath the skin. It is a discolored area of skin, usually blue, purple, or black at first, gradually fading to yellow before disappearing entirely after about a week. The bruise turns yellow as a result of the breakdown of hemoglobin in red blood cells.

How to treat a bruise

1 Leave the bruise alone. Do not rub or massage it.

2 Apply an ice pack for about 10 minutes immediately after the injury to reduce the area of bruising.

3 If a leg is bruised, rest with the feet propped up.

BURNS AND SCALDS

Minor burns and scalds damage only the top layer of skin over a fairly small area, causing reddening and, sometimes, blistering. These injuries can be treated at home. More serious burns that damage larger areas and penetrate the skin deeply require professional care (see SEVERE BURNS, page 133).

Superficial burns usually heal fairly rapidly, and the damaged layer of skin may peel away after several days. However, burns can be extremely painful, and first-aid treatment is therefore directed primarily at relieving pain.

Minor SUNBURN (page 140) is a common example of a superficial burn.

How to treat a minor burn

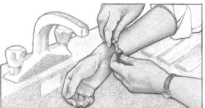

1 Immerse the burned area in cold, preferably running, water or apply a cold water compress until the pain subsides.

2 Remove constricting items, such as watches, belts, or rings, from the burned area in case swelling occurs.

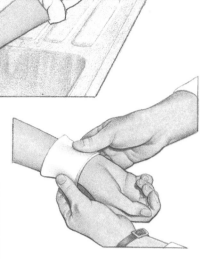

3 Do not prick any blisters that have formed or apply any lotions or creams. Lightly bandage the burned area with a clean, dry gauze or cloth dressing. Do not use anything fluffy that might stick to the burn.

CUTS AND SCRAPES

Bleeding from minor cuts and scrapes usually stops on its own within a short time as the blood clots. If bleeding does not stop, press a clean, nonfluffy pad (not cotton) over the wound for a few minutes.

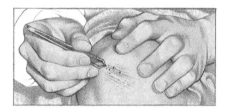

1 If the wound has dirt in it, rinse it under the faucet, using lukewarm water; then extract any dirt particles with tweezers.

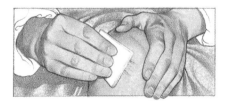

2 Dry the cut or scrape by patting gently with sterile gauze (not with fluffy cotton).

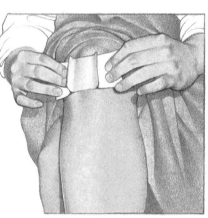

3 Cover the cut or scrape with an adhesive bandage of an appropriate size (longer than the wound).

When to see your doctor

Consult your doctor if the wound becomes tender, inflamed, or infected; if it is very deep; if it is on the face; if it is more than ¹/₂ inch (1 cm) long and gaping so that it may need stitching to prevent scarring; if it is very dirty; if it is a deep puncture wound from a nail or an animal's tooth; or if you experience numbness, tingling, or weakness in an affected arm or leg.

DENTAL INJURY

If a tooth is fractured by a direct blow or a fall onto a hard surface, make an appointment immediately with your dentist. If bacteria enter the tooth, they can cause infection and loss of the tooth.

It is even more important to act swiftly if a tooth has been completely knocked out of its socket. Called an "avulsed" tooth, it may reattach itself to the bone if it is splinted by a dentist within 2 hours.

Take aspirin to ease the pain, but do not place an aspirin directly on the gums or a damaged tooth.

How to treat an avulsed tooth

1 Clean the tooth with a rinse of water or saliva.

2 Gently replace the tooth in its socket.

3 Hold the tooth in place with your finger or by biting onto a handkerchief.

4 Go to your dentist, who will splint the tooth to give it time to become reimplanted.

FAINTNESS AND FAINTING

Fainting is a temporary loss of consciousness that occurs when not enough oxygen reaches the brain. It can be caused by standing still for long periods of time or by getting up too quickly. It can also be brought on by severe pain, stress, or fear.

If someone has fainted, first check that breathing is normal. Lay the person on his or her back, with legs raised above the level of the head. Hold the legs up or rest them on a chair. Loosen any tight clothing, such as a shirt collar or waistband. If you are indoors, open a window to let plenty of fresh air circulate. If you are outside, make sure the person is not in the sun. Do not allow the person to get up for a few minutes after regaining consciousness.

If you feel faint: Lie down with your legs raised. If this is not possible, sit with your head bent between your knees until you feel better.

FOREIGN BODY IN EYE

A foreign body on the surface of the eye can cause pain, redness, and sensitivity to light. The foreign body often causes uncontrollable watering and blinking. Although these symptoms may lessen even if the foreign body remains on the eye, the object must be removed to prevent infection, which can cause blindness.

Any foreign body that has penetrated the eye should be removed by an ophthalmologist. To prevent the person from rubbing the eye, cover both eyes with soft pads, bandaging them lightly in place by wrapping a clean length of gauze around the victim's head. On the way to the hospital, keep the victim in a prone position.

Superficial foreign bodies (such as eyelashes or specks of dirt) that are on the white of the eye or the inside of the eyelid may be removed at home.

How to remove a foreign body from the eye

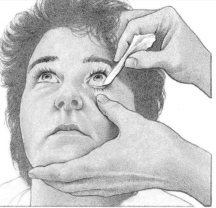

1 Wash your hands and seat the individual in good light. Ask him or her to look up while you gently pull the lower lid down. If you can see the foreign body, try picking it off with the moistened corner of a clean cloth.

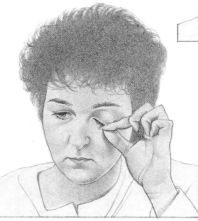

2 If you cannot see the object, gently pull the upper lid down and forward over the lower lid and let it slide back. This motion may be enough to dislodge the foreign body.

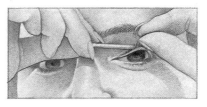

3 If the object remains in place, ask the person to look down while you place a matchstick across the upper lid and fold the lid up over the match. If you can see the object, pick it off with the moistened corner of a clean cloth.

4 If all attempts are unsuccessful, lightly cover the eye with a soft pad and seek medical help.

FRACTURES AND DISLOCATIONS

It is not always possible, without an X-ray, to tell whether a bone is broken. You should suspect a dislocation or fracture if the victim cannot move or put weight on the injured part or if it is very painful or looks obviously misshapen.

Do not try to replace a dislocated joint yourself. This should be done only by a doctor or other trained professional. Splint the dislocated limb in the position in which you found it or, in the case of a dislocated shoulder, apply a sling.

A person with a suspected fracture or dislocation should be taken to the hospital. If walking is impossible, call for medical help.

First aid for a fracture

1 Treat any serious BLEEDING (page 133), trying to move the victim as little as possible.

2 Do not give the person anything to eat or drink in case a general anesthetic is required. If the victim cannot be moved, keep him or her warm and watch for signs of SHOCK (page 132) while you wait for a doctor or other professional help to arrive.

HEAD INJURIES

Wounds on the scalp almost always bleed profusely. A superficial wound can be treated by covering it with a clean pad and applying steady pressure. If you suspect a serious head injury, tie the pad lightly over the wound, being very careful not to press too hard. This will ensure that you do not push any foreign bodies or pieces of broken skull into the brain. If a clear fluid trickles out of the ear, place a clean pad over the affected ear and lay the victim down on that side to encourage drainage of the fluid from the ear. If the fluid drains out of the nose, turn the victim on his or her side and call out for someone to get medical help.

APPLYING A SPLINT

If you must move the victim or if you have to wait a long time for medical help, he or she will probably be more comfortable if you immobilize the broken part by splinting it.

Broken leg

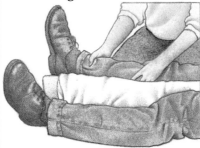

1 Place padding between the two legs, and carefully move the uninjured leg toward the one that has been injured.

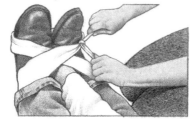

2 Apply a figure-of-eight bandage around the ankles and tie it as securely as possible.

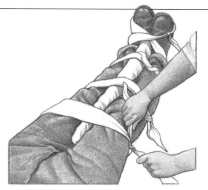

3 Tie the legs together in several places, taking care to avoid the site of the fracture.

Broken lower arm

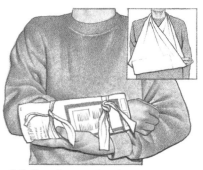

1 Splint the arm in a bent position across the chest, using anything rigid, and tie it in at least two places near (not on) the site of injury.

2 Support the arm in a sling, making sure the fingers are slightly higher than the elbow.

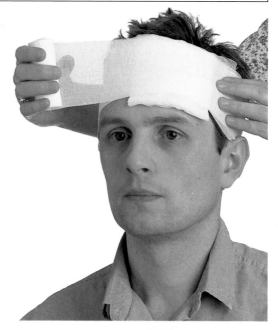

Dressing a head wound
Place a sterile dressing or any clean pad over the wound, use two or three turns of a roller bandage to hold the dressing, then secure with safety pins.

NOSEBLEEDS

Bleeding from the nose is common and is not usually a cause for concern. Causes include minor injury to the nose, blowing the nose repeatedly, or picking the nose. Very dry houses also can lead to nosebleeds.

If you have a nosebleed, sit down and lean forward slightly. Breathe through the mouth and pinch both nostrils firmly for about 15 minutes. This encourages the formation of a blood clot, which will seal the damaged blood vessels. The nostrils should then be released slowly. Avoid blowing your nose for several hours after bleeding has stopped, as this may dislodge the blood clot.

Get medical help if you suspect the nose is broken, if bleeding continues for more than 20 minutes, or if bleeding follows a blow to the head (this could indicate a fractured skull).

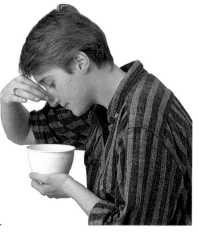

SLIVERS

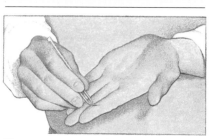

To remove a small sliver that projects from the skin, grasp the end of it with a pair of tweezers and pull gently. If the sliver has become completely embedded in the skin, sterilize the sharp end of a needle by holding it in a flame for a few seconds; then slit the skin over the sliver and lift it up with the needle tip. You should now be able to grasp the sliver with tweezers. If it does not come out easily, seek medical help.

POISONOUS PLANTS

Some types of plants can cause an allergic reaction if your skin comes in contact with the leaves. The most common of these plants in the US are poison ivy, poison oak, and poison sumac.

If you come into contact with a poisonous plant:

1 Wash the affected area with soap and water, rub with alcohol, and apply calamine lotion.

2 Wash any clothing that has come into contact with the plant.

3 Consult your doctor if you have a severe reaction.

Poison sumac

Poison ivy

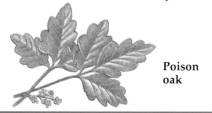

Poison oak

SEIZURES

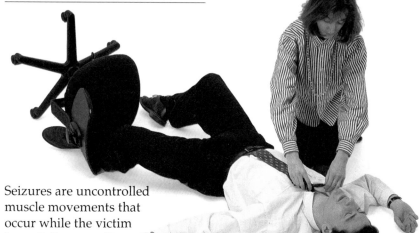

Seizures are uncontrolled muscle movements that occur while the victim is partially or totally unconscious. Seizures result from a temporary disturbance in the brain's electrical activity. Although they are alarming to witness, they usually end within a few minutes. When a person has a major (grand mal) epileptic seizure, he or she loses consciousness and the entire body stiffens and then twitches uncontrollably. Bowel and bladder control may be temporarily lost. Always call a doctor if the seizure lasts longer than 5 minutes or if a second seizure begins.

What to do

1 Clear away any furniture or objects from the area so the person is not in danger of physical injury. Do not try to restrain the person's movements and do not put anything into the mouth.

2 Loosen tight clothing around the person's neck.

3 Once jerking movements have stopped, wait for the person to regain consciousness and then find a quiet place for him or her to rest.

SPRAIN

The most commonly sprained joint is the ankle, usually as a result of "rolling over" on the outside of the foot.

A sudden pull of this kind can stretch or tear the ligaments that help support the ankle joint. The fibrous capsule (bursa) that encloses the joint may also be damaged.

A sprain causes painful swelling of the joint, which cannot be moved without increasing the pain. A severe sprain may be indistinguishable from a fracture. If you are in doubt, treat the injury as a FRACTURE (page 138).

First aid for a sprained ankle

1 The person may not be able to move the affected joint or even put weight on it. Help him or her into a comfortable position and apply a cold compress for 30 minutes.

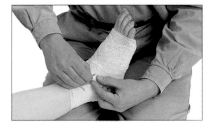

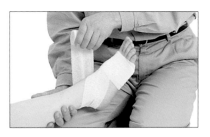

2 Cover with a pad. Secure it with a bandage, making two turns around the foot. Bring the bandage across the top and around the ankle.

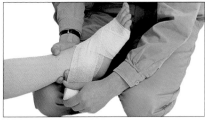

3 Continue bandaging in figures-of-eight, with each turn of the bandage overlapping the previous turn by three quarters of its width.

4 Continue bandaging until the foot (not the toes), ankle, and lower leg are covered. Secure the loose end. Seek medical aid.

STRAIN

Tearing or stretching a muscle as a result of suddenly overloading it may result in bleeding into the muscles, pain, swelling, and muscle spasm. Strain of the muscles in the lower back, for example, is a very common cause of back pain.

Strains are most common among athletes. The risk of suffering a strain can be reduced by performing warm-up exercises before you begin any sports activity.

First-aid treatment for a strain consists mainly of making the person as comfortable as possible and giving aspirin (children under 16 should *not* take aspirin) or acetaminophen.

First aid for a muscle strain

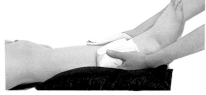

1 Apply an ice pack or cold compress to reduce pain and swelling. Analgesics (painkillers) may also be taken for pain relief.

2 An injured limb should be rested in a raised position for 48 hours. If you have a strained back, rest lying down until the pain diminishes.

3 After resting the muscle for 48 hours, physical therapy should be started as soon as possible to prevent any long-term damage.

SUNBURN

Sunburn is caused by overexposure to the ultraviolet rays of the sun. The skin may become red and tender and may blister. Exposure over long periods can lead to skin cancer.

Treating sunburn

1 Apply a cream to soothe the skin. If it is very painful, call a doctor.

2 Avoid further exposure to the sun, unless you are fully clothed.

How to prevent sunburn

1 Expose yourself gradually to the sun; avoid the midday sun.

2 Use a sunscreen with a high protection factor.

FAMILY HEALTH RECORD

Keep a record of important medical information. You can make a photocopy of this chart for each family member.

Name _____ Date of birth _____

Name and telephone number of doctor(s) _____

Blood type _____ Allergies _____

IMMUNIZATIONS

Diphtheria, pertussis, tetanus (DPT)		Poliomyelitis		Measles, mumps, rubella		Other immunizations	
Age usually administered	Date of vaccine	Age usually administered	Date of vaccine	Age usually administered	Date of vaccine	Types	Date of vaccine
2 months 4 months 6 months 18 months 4–6 years		2 months 4 months 18 months 4–6 years		15 months			

MAJOR ILLNESSES/SURGERY   Date   Treatment/outcome

MEDICATIONS   Date started   Date stopped

CHECKUPS/TESTS   Date/result   Date/result   Date/result

	Date/result	Date/result	Date/result
Blood pressure Blood cholesterol Dental examination Cervical (Pap) smear Mammogram Eye examination			

INDEX

Page numbers in *italics* refer to illustrations and captions.

Photograph sources:

Colorific Photo Library **14**
Jaqui Farrow/Bubbles **29**
The Image Bank **102** (center); **111** (top); **111** (center)
Institute of Dermatology **89** (top); **90** (top and bottom)
Camilla Jessel **27** (top right)
Dr Paul Myers **91** (center)
National Medical Slide Bank **55** (top); **93** (top left); **93** (top right); **93** (center right); **93** (bottom left); **93** (bottom right)
The Photo Co-op **52**
Photographers' Library **12** (bottom)
Pictor International **9**; **115** (bottom right); **116** (center)
Barry Richards (National Heart Hospital) **76**
Dr Hugh Rushton/Dr Philip Kingsley **116** (top)
Science Photo Library **42**; **55** (center); **78** (center); **82**; **84** (center); **85**; **88** (bottom right); **89** (bottom); **99** (bottom left); **113** (bottom left)
Howard Sochurek **77** (bottom)

Spectrum Colour Library **129**
Sporting Pictures (UK) **60**
Tony Stone Worldwide **113** (top) and front cover
Dr Ian Williams **43**; **90** (top)
Zefa Picture Library **107**; **115** (bottom left)

Commissioned photography:
Steve Bartholomew
Stephan Oliver
Susanna Price
Clive Streeter

Illustrators:
David Ashby
Russell Barnet
Karen Cochrane
Graham Corbett
David Fathers
Tony Graham
Chris Jenkins

Kevin Jones Assoc.
Coral Mula
Gilly Newman
Lynda Payne
Howard Pemberton
Andrew Popkiewicz
James Robbins
Lydia Umney
John Woodcock

Charts:
Technical Art Services

Airbrushing:
Janos Marffy
Roy Flooks

Health campaign posters on pages 18–20 courtesy of:

American Medical Association **18** (top left); Central Office of Information, UK **19** (bottom right); Department of Transport, UK **18** (bottom left); Health Education Authority, UK **19** (top left); Kaufmännische Krankenkasse, West-Germany **18** (top right); National Consumer Agency of Denmark/ Freddy Milton **19** (top center); Project Icarus, UK **20** (center)